W9-DFE-882

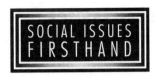

Performance-
Enhancing Drugs

Other Books in the Social Issues Firsthand Series:

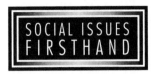

Performance-Enhancing Drugs

Norah Piehl, Book Editor

GREENHAVEN PRESS
A part of Gale, Cengage Learning

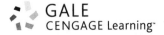
GALE
CENGAGE Learning™

Detroit • New York • San Francisco • New Haven, Conn • Waterville, Maine • London

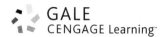

Christine Nasso, *Publisher*
Elizabeth Des Chenes, *Managing Editor*

© 2010 Greenhaven Press, a part of Gale, Cengage Learning.

Gale and Greenhaven Press are registered trademarks used herein under license.

For more information, contact:
Greenhaven Press
27500 Drake Rd.
Farmington Hills, MI 48331-3535
Or you can visit our Internet site at gale.cengage.com

For product information and technology assistance, contact us at

Gale Customer Support, 1-800-877-4253
For permission to use material from this text or product, submit all requests online at www.cengage.com/permissions

Further permissions questions can be emailed to permissionrequest@cengage.com

Articles in Greenhaven Press anthologies are often edited for length to meet page requirements. In addition, original titles of these works are changed to clearly present the main thesis and to explicitly indicate the author's opinion. Every effort is made to ensure that Greenhaven Press accurately reflects the original intent of the authors. Every effort has been made to trace the owners of copyrighted material.

LIBRARY OF CONGRESS CATALOGING-IN-PUBLICATION DATA

Performace-enhancing drugs / Norah Piehl, book editor.
    p. cm. -- Social issues firsthand
Includes bibliographical references and index.
ISBN 978-0-7377-5011-9 (hardcover)
    1. Athletes--Drug use. 2. Anabolic steroids--Health aspects. 3. Doping in sports.
I. Piehl, Norah.
    RC1230.P4764 2010
    362.29--dc22
                                                    2010004544

Printed in the United States of America
1 2 3 4 5 6 7 14 13 12 11 10

Contents

Professional cyclist Patrik Sinkewitz was banned from the Tour de France after testing positive for testosterone. In this interview, he discusses the prevalence of doping and his own attitudes toward drug use, regulation, and enforcement.

Chapter 3: Performance-Enhancing Drugs Outside the Arena

Foreword

Social issues are often viewed in abstract terms. Pressing challenges such as poverty, homelessness, and addiction are viewed as problems to be defined and solved. Politicians, social scientists, and other experts engage in debates about the extent of the problems, their causes, and how best to remedy them. Often overlooked in these discussions is the human dimension of the issue. Behind every policy debate over poverty, homelessness, and substance abuse, for example, are real people struggling to make ends meet, to survive life on the streets, and to overcome addiction to drugs and alcohol. Their stories are ubiquitous and compelling. They are the stories of everyday people—perhaps your own family members or friends—and yet they rarely influence the debates taking place in state capitols, the national Congress, or the courts.

The disparity between the public debate and private experience of social issues is well illustrated by looking at the topic of poverty. Each year the U.S. Census Bureau establishes a poverty threshold. A household with an income below the threshold is defined as poor, while a household with an income above the threshold is considered able to live on a basic subsistence level. For example, in 2003 a family of two was considered poor if its income was less than $12,015; a family of four was defined as poor if its income was less than $18,810. Based on this system, the bureau estimates that 35.9 million Americans (12.5 percent of the population) lived below the poverty line in 2003, including 12.9 million children below the age of eighteen.

Commentators disagree about what these statistics mean. Social activists insist that the huge number of officially poor Americans translates into human suffering. Even many families that have incomes above the threshold, they maintain, are likely to be struggling to get by. Other commentators insist that the statistics exaggerate the problem of poverty in the United States. Compared to people in developing countries, they point out, most so-called poor families have a high quality of life. As stated by journalist Fidelis Iyebote, "Cars are owned by 70 percent of 'poor' households. . . . Color televisions belong to 97 percent of the 'poor' [and] videocassette recorders belong to nearly 75 percent. . . . Sixty-four percent have microwave ovens, half own a stereo system, and over a quarter possess an automatic dishwasher."

However, this debate over the poverty threshold and what it means is likely irrelevant to a person living in poverty. Simply put, poor people do not need the government to tell them whether they are poor. They can see it in the stack of bills they cannot pay. They are aware of it when they are forced to choose between paying rent or buying food for their children. They become painfully conscious of it when they lose their homes and are forced to live in their cars or on the streets. Indeed, the written stories of poor people define the meaning of poverty more vividly than a government bureaucracy could ever hope to. Narratives composed by the poor describe losing jobs due to injury or mental illness, depict horrific tales of childhood abuse and spousal violence, recount the loss of friends and family members. They evoke the slipping away of social supports and government assistance, the descent into substance abuse and addiction, the harsh realities of life on the streets. These are the perspectives on poverty that are too often omitted from discussions over the extent of the problem and how to solve it.

Greenhaven Press's *Social Issues Firsthand* series provides a forum for the often-overlooked human perspectives on society's most divisive topics of debate. Each volume focuses on one social issue and presents a collection of ten to sixteen narratives by those who have had personal involvement with the topic. Extra care has been taken to include a diverse range of perspectives. For example, in the volume on adoption, readers will find the stories of birth parents who have made an adoption plan, adoptive parents, and adoptees themselves. After exposure to these varied points of view, the reader will have a clearer understanding that adoption is an intense, emotional experience full of joyous highs and painful lows for all concerned.

The debate surrounding embryonic stem cell research illustrates the moral and ethical pressure that the public brings to bear on the scientific community. However, while nonexperts often criticize scientists for not considering the potential negative impact of their work, ironically the public's reaction against such discoveries can produce harmful results as well. For example, although the outcry against embryonic stem cell research in the United States has resulted in fewer embryos being destroyed, those with Parkinson's, such as actor Michael J. Fox, have argued that prohibiting the development of new stem cell lines ultimately will prevent a timely cure for the disease that is killing Fox and thousands of others.

Each book in the series contains several features that enhance its usefulness, including an in-depth introduction, an annotated table of contents, bibliographies for further research, a list of organizations to contact, and a thorough index. These elements—combined with the poignant voices of people touched by tragedy and triumph—make the *Social Issues Firsthand* series a valuable resource for research on today's topics of political discussion.

Introduction

During the 2008 Summer Olympics, millions of people worldwide tuned their televisions to coverage of the games, in large part to see whether American swimmer Michael Phelps would achieve his much-hyped quest for eight gold medals. Even as Phelps chased his dream (ultimately successfully), breaking several Olympic and world records in the process, other swimmers were also shattering world records in the Beijing National Aquatics Center, known as the Water Cube.

Swimming world records had been dropping like flies since earlier in 2008, when many of the world's top competitive swimmers adopted Speedo's LZR Racer Suit, marketed as "the world's fastest swimsuit." The nearly full-body suit, which had been developed after extensive high-tech testing, was designed to make the swimmer's body as hydrodynamic and streamlined as possible while increasing buoyancy and reducing drag in the water. In the first two seasons following the suit's introduction in February 2008, ninety-three world records were broken by swimmers wearing the suit, and thirty-three of the thirty-six Olympic medals for swimming in 2008 (including all eight of Phelps's) were won by swimmers wearing the LZR Racer.

In July 2009, however, just a little less than a year after Phelps's historic achievement, swimming's governing body, Fédération Internationale de Natation (FINA), reversed a previous decision and voted to ban high-tech suits like the LZR beginning in January 2010. Although all those recent world records will stand, swimmers acknowledge that, following the ban, it may be a very long time before world records are broken again. "A lot of us are joking that this might be the fastest we ever go," American backstroke specialist Aaron Peirsol told the Associated Press after the ban was announced. "We might as well enjoy this year."

In a previous statement about high-tech suits like the LZR Racer, FINA asserted its position that "the main and core principle is that swimming is a sport essentially based on the physical performance of the athlete." Contentions like this form the backbone of many arguments around the legality and ethics of various sorts of performance enhancement. Journalists, bioethicists, and philosophers of sport look at this issue from various perspectives, but in many cases, the question comes down to this: what are sports designed to measure, and how do various methods of performance enhancement affect (or not affect) that measurement? Considering questions like this can highlight the often-blurred line between forms of performance enhancement that are socially, legally, and ethically acceptable—even admired—and those that are looked down on or banned outright.

Taken in the broadest terms, some of the most basic principles of an athletic lifestyle can be considered forms of performance enhancement, even though no one would argue against them. Eating a balanced diet—even a specialized nutrition plan developed in conjunction with professional nutritionists—and following a training plan—even a sophisticated, demanding regimen overseen by professional trainers and coaches—are widely seen as essential aspects of sports excellence.

Yet, as absurd as it might sound, these activities could nonetheless be broadly categorized with some other, more ethically questionable, forms of performance enhancement. An athlete who sticks to a specially designed diet and follows a strict training schedule in advance of a competition would be expected to outperform one who sits in front of the television and eats potato chips all day, regardless of their individual innate physical skills or athletic ability. Since our society values both those athletes who exhibit natural superiority and those who achieve their skills—at least in part—through training, hard work, and dedication, performance enhancement through diet and exercise does not violate what we hope to measure in sports competitions.

Clearly this type of performance enhancement through training and diet is considered exemplary, even essential, to the "spirit of sport," one of the three criteria laid out by the World Anti-Doping Code to evaluate the ethics of various modes of performance enhancement. Things become more complicated, however, when we start to consider enhancements made possible by equipment and other forms of technology. The recent controversy surrounding the LZR Racer swimsuit is only the latest in a long series of debates about the ethics of sporting equipment and other high-tech innovations. Issues surrounding these high-tech enhancements are not quite as clear-cut as those regarding diet and training.

In his article, "Rethinking Enhancement in Sport," Andy Miah helpfully differentiates among various types of technological enhancement. Some, like helmets in football and supportive shoes in running, are designed as much to improve safety as to enhance performance, and pose few, if any, ethical quandaries. Others, such as redesigned golf clubs that provide far greater stroke accuracy or cycling handlebars and helmets that promote greatly increased aerodynamics, begin to blur the line. Often, the decision lies in the answer to the following question: who is accomplishing the feat of athletic skill, the athlete or her equipment? Most often, rules governing particular sports weigh in on this issue by mandating standards for equipment: the size of catcher's mitts, the weight and composition of javelins, and so forth. This means that when technology starts to jump ahead of existing sports rules—as in the case of the LZR Racer suit or the composition of archery bows, barbells, bicycles, and so on, sports governing bodies need to be prepared to adapt accordingly and to consider each new innovation's effects on a particular sport, its participants, and its fans.

The most ethically complex areas are those in which technological enhancements seem to cross the line into the realm of physical modifications to athletes' own bodies. Most people, if asked about their response to performance-enhancing drug use by athletes, would express disapproval or disgust at the practice, even if they could not explain exactly why the idea is so distasteful. In his book, *The Case Against Perfection*, Michael J. Sandel argues that physical enhancements—such as those achieved by blood doping, the use of steroids, and so forth—risk turning sport into spectacle. He uses the example of Major League Baseball's home run derby, held in conjunction with the annual All-Star Game: "A game in which . . . sluggers routinely hit home runs might be amusing for a time, but it would lack the human drama and complexity of baseball, in which even the greatest hitters fail more often than they succeed."

Technology is enabling professional athletes—not to mention aspiring amateurs—to overcome some of their bodies' natural limitations. Ethicists often point to the example of golfer Tiger Woods, who started routinely winning major golf tournaments shortly after having his vision corrected through laser eye surgery. Others point to the ethically debatable practice of athletes sleeping in hypoxic tents to simulate the low-oxygen conditions at high altitudes. This process "naturally" increases athletes' red blood cell count, thereby achieving exactly the same result as those who engage in illegal blood doping by taking the drug known as EPO (erythropoietin) that also increases red blood cell count. Why is a high-tech solution like a hypoxic tent acceptable to the World Anti-Doping Agency when the use of performance-enhancing drugs that achieve the same ends is not?

Where do we draw the line between technological innovations like hypoxic tents and buoyancy-improving swimsuits and the use of banned substances? Like many ethical questions, it is not simply a matter of "following the rules," especially when scientists and engineers are continually developing new products faster than sports can possibly adjudicate on them. These questions are only likely to grow more complicated, as genetic modifications to athletes' own bodies become less a topic for science fiction and more a reality that elite athletes, coaches, government agencies, and sports-governing bodies will need to grapple with. The ethical questions surrounding performance enhancement in athletics are likely to gain complexity—and importance—as technology helps push the boundaries of what the human body can achieve.

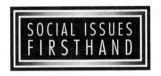

CHAPTER 1

Performance-Enhancing Drugs in Sports

Riding Under the Influence

Joe Parkin

In the late 1980s and early 1990s, Joe Parkin spent six seasons on the professional cycling circuit in Belgium. As he relates in his memoir, A Dog in a Hat, *the cutthroat, physically exhausting world of European professional cycling was very different from the competitions in which Parkin had excelled when he was an amateur cyclist in California.*

Along with grueling schedules and physically demanding competitions, Parkin also encountered the underground but widely accepted culture of performance-enhancing drugs. Parkin not only relates the riders' and team managers' casual attitude toward the drugs but also graphically recounts the extreme measures to which riders went to avoid detection.

Joe Parkin was one of the first Americans to become a professional bicycle racer in Europe. He represented the United States at the World Professional Road Cycling Championships, the World Professional Cyclocross Championships, and the World Professional Mountain Bike Championships. He currently writes about cycling issues on his blog: 6 Years in a Rain Cape (www.6yearsinaraincape.com).

My parents came to visit me in the spring and were able to catch the Brabantse Pijl (Flèche Brabanconne in Flemish) and the Three Days of de Panne [cycling races]. My dad, who traveled often for work, had amassed enough frequent-flyer miles to allow them to fly first class to London. After a night in London they took the ferry from Dover across the water to Oostende, where I picked them up. I had been able to find them a new little hotel in the neighboring town of Aalter. Having them come was a mixed blessing. On the one hand, they were my parents, and I wanted them to see me in my element. On the other hand, I was having a hard time finding my element that year. Nonetheless, I was anxious to have my dad see the races, since he was more skeptical and less appreciative of my career than my mom.

Entertaining friends and family while you're trying to race is difficult in every situation, but we had the added hurdles of language, culture, and undiagnosed illness. Not long after this trip, my dad was diagnosed with Alzheimer's disease. He was already displaying many of the symptoms, but his young age of 52 kept doctors from making the correct evaluation. My mom was nearing her wits' end; in fact, she had been hovering in that area for some time before their trip. My dad had been having a hard time speaking for a while, and most of our conversations were one-sided, with him mostly just agreeing with whatever my mom and I had said. I think she had already learned to speak on his behalf to a great extent.

I'd been able to borrow an old Audi 80 from a friend for my parents' visit because I still didn't have my own car. I used Albert's car on occasion and had driven various team box vans back from races when he'd decided to have a few beers before we left, so I was familiar with the Belgian roads and style of driving. My dad was scared to death when I was behind the wheel, and before each trip he'd ask if he could drive instead.

I was able to make it to the start of the Brabantse Pijl without killing anyone and left my mom and dad to fend for themselves while I got dressed with the rest of the team. The weather was near perfect for April in Belgium, so it should have been a good race for me to find the finish. I wasn't riding well enough to finish with a great result, but I didn't see any reason why I couldn't ride well enough to make myself happy.

"Something Extra"

Albert and my director, Patrick Versluys, thought otherwise; they thought this was the perfect opportunity for me to do something extra, especially now that my parents had arrived. I was handed two Captagon wrapped in aluminum foil and instructed to take one before the start and one if I felt I was going to make it into the final. Captagon is the brand name for fenethylline, a stimulant that affects the body in a way similar to amphetamine. I didn't know exactly what it was, but I did know it was on the doping list, and I had heard teammates talk about it as somewhat weak. Nevertheless, they spoke of it in the same breath as the hard-core amphetamines. If it had been some sort of caffeine concoction or even a pill for late-race cramps, I would have non-chalantly slid the goods into my jersey pocket. But this was different. I winced in protest.

"I don't know," I whined. "There's control here."

They didn't care about the doping control. If I were picked to be tested after the race, they'd find a way around my getting caught. I didn't feel like raising the clean-bike-racer flag, so I stuffed the drugs into my pocket. The European teams of that era (in Belgium especially) didn't think highly of goody-two-shoes riders. Like the vaunted Blue Code of Silence among police, pro bike racing definitely had the Lycra Code of Silence. I suspect that code is still strong today.

As an American I stuck out enough, so I didn't need to give anybody cause for concern, especially as poorly as I was riding. Many of the team managers, teammates, friends, and fans I had while living in Belgium would have looked at *not* taking the drugs as a failure to give 100 percent to being a cyclist, and I didn't want to suddenly find myself left at home for every race because I openly refused to try. I got back on my bike and rolled over to my mom and dad.

Not My First Time

I was now faced with a decision: Eat the Captagon as prescribed and most likely ride well but risk the doping control, or forget it and hope for the best. I was a conscientious objector and willful abstainer, but I was not a drug virgin, which made the decision a bit more difficult. The year before I had made the split in a small semiclassic in the Ardennes. I wasn't riding well, and I was feeling even worse. My stomach was killing me, and the tempo in the group was not helping matters. I was fighting with the bike for all I was worth, wishing I had never made it into this stupid front group. The team car showed up to find out how I was feeling. Usually I was able to muster some kind of casual complaint about a specific issue, but this time "I feel shitty" and "stomach" were the only words I could form. I was handed a small bottle, about half the size of a half-pint hip flask for booze and made of plastic.

"This will help," Florent told me. "Not too much—just half now, half later if you want it."

Part of me wanted to believe that those guys somehow had a small pharmacy on board that would fix my stomach. Most of me knew I was getting ready to take off my party dress. I yanked out the cork with my teeth in a style that has been passed down through generations of my hard-drinking ancestors and drank from the flask. I tasted Coca-Cola, Champ (a syrupy sugar drink), and something chalky. Maybe they had just given me something for my stomach after all, I thought. My tongue pushed the chalky particles out from between my teeth as I rode back toward the front of the group. The Coke was helping my stomach.

A New Perspective

The temperature was in the middle to upper 70s, warm by Belgian standards, but goose bumps were beginning to form on my legs along with a strange sheen from the sweat that looked like baby oil to me. My position on the bike went from hunched over and fighting to upright and relaxed. Within minutes after I had consumed half of the little flask, I was riding at the front of the group, climbing with my hands resting comfortably on the top of the handlebars, close to the stem. It felt as if the tempo had slowed, and I looked back to see what was going on. I felt that someone would surely be attacking at any moment because the pace was so slow. I looked back again. Many of the other riders in the group were fighting with their bikes, as I had been doing just a few minutes before.

"What is wrong with these people?" I wondered out loud to myself.

If we continued riding so slowly, I was sure we were going to get caught. I started upping the tempo, ever so slightly. We approached the finishing circuits, so I knocked back the rest of the contents of the flask. I made sure to put the thing back in my pocket instead of throwing it to the side of the road. I didn't want anyone to sample the contents. After the finish line and some right and left turns, there was a short climb out of town. On the first passage of this climb I made sure to position myself toward the front and then fought back the urge to take the lead. On the second climb of the same hill, I was no longer able to control my energy. I went to the lead and set the tempo. I looked back as former Tour de France stage winners, classics winners, and other notable bike racers were put into trouble by the pace. All the while I was sitting comfortably on my bike, practically breathing through my nose.

When we made it to a lap and a half to go, Corneille Daems made an offer to the seven or eight riders still in the breakaway for him to win the race. I cannot remember the amount he proposed, but it was pretty good, good enough for most of the rest of them. But I was feeling too strong.

"*Non.*" I waved him off. "*Nee.*" After one or two more turns through the pace line Edwig van Hooydonk approached me, pushing his freckled face toward mine.

"You want to win?" he asked accusingly and shot me a glare as if I had just asked to sleep with his wife.

"*Ja,*" I answered. But we were cut short as Daems attacked and the rest of the group chased him.

A Dog with a Hat On

I had heard a lot of the old Belgians use the expression, *"een hond met een hoed op,"* which means "a dog with a hat on." In the context in which I heard it, I took it to mean that you see a dog in a hat when a normal situation changes, when something looks out of place. When instructing a young rider to control the race by reacting early and often to other teams' attacks, a director might tell the rider to look for a dog with a hat on.

In my state, I could see the hat before the dog even decided to put it on. In fact, I could see what color underwear the dog was wearing. I'm pretty sure Superman could leap tall buildings and see through walls and all that because he was jacked to the gills on amphetamine. I was countering my competitors' attacks even before they thought about making them. I was inflicting excruciating pain on every inch of my body, but I didn't care. It was amazing!

Unfortunately, each of my new strengths was outweighed by the fact that I was also becoming more stupid by the second. In reacting to my competitors before they could even attack, I was doing more work than I needed to. I was controlling the race in such a way that it was actually easier on them. If we'd been racing in Las Vegas, I would have been the drunk at the poker game trying to go all-in on a pair of twos after showing everyone else my cards.

Increasing Clarity

Van Hooydonk attacked and went clear. He won. I studied the situation and somehow figured out that I was no longer going to win and, that being the case, should stay off the podium to lessen the odds of being sent to doping control. Most medical controls are limited to the top three riders, plus two random picks. Usually the rest of the top 10 finishers are not included in the random selection and this race was no exception.

I was still supernatural well into the night. I was up early the next morning and went to ride off my hangover. Plodding along at a slow speed was about all I could handle, so I stayed perched on my bike for most of the day. The day after that I went to a kermis race [a short, closed-circuit race]. I can't remember if this was one I was supposed to ride or if I thought it would be good to blow the legs out a bit, but the extra effort I had been able to expend a couple days before had taken its toll. I am sure it was partly perception, since the race had come so easily when I was doped, but as well as I knew my body, I knew I had done a good job of hurting it.

A doctor once told me that a well-trained athlete can find about 85 percent of his potential, whereas a well-trained athlete on amphetamines will be able to perform at 105 percent. Whether or not that could be proven didn't matter to me because I was feeling the aftereffects in this kermis race. I dropped out at about the two-hour mark, determined that this was going to be the last time I would feel this way.

Looking My Parents in the Face

As I waited for the start of the Brabantse Pijl, the ill effects of the doping the year before were mostly sequestered in the far recesses of my mind. Instead, I remembered being Superman. Still, I didn't want anything to do with the Captagon tablets. If I had a saving grace, it was the fear of being the first American to get popped for doping. I couldn't stand the thought. Perhaps it was a weak crutch, but it was the one I was leaning on, and it worked for me. I also thought about how the doping controls were being beaten at the time: catheters filling the rider's bladder with "clean" urine or modified condoms placed in other orifices and then filled with "clean" urine. Those were the two that stuck out, but there were a host of others.

I could almost see a bad television sitcom flashback scene, with me lying on a table wearing a former Kentucky Derby winner's victory wreath while a fat Belgian soigneur [trainer] helped get me ready to beat the control. After a loud knock a blond stripper dressed like a nurse would appear and open the door. My parents would be standing on the other side, hoping to come in and congratulate me on my win.

"Oh, hi," the nurse would say, giggling and pointing at me. "Joe can't come to the door right now 'cause that fat man is shoving a condom in his butt. Hee hee."

Imaginary sitcom nightmare or not, I didn't want to see the expressions on my parents' faces or feel the pain on mine. About halfway through the Brabantse Pijl, I knew I was not going to take the pill I had been supposed to take at the start. A little while later, after struggling with the decision to avoid the second pill as well, I realized that I wasn't paying attention to the race at all. In fact, I was no longer in the first group. On the second or third finishing circuits, I turned left and headed for the showers.

I looked my bosses in the eyes and told them that what they had given me hadn't worked and, in fact, had blocked my legs. For some reason they bought it. More importantly, I was able to meet my parents' eyes when I explained that it just hadn't been my day. At that moment in time, looking them in the face while they felt sorry for me was better than staring at their shoes while they offered their congratulations.

Why Mcgwire Won't Get My Vote

Ann Killion

In the summer of 1998, die-hard and casual baseball fans alike were glued to their television screens and radios as two beloved players—Mark McGwire of the St. Louis Cardinals and Sammy Sosa of the Chicago Cubs—battled to break Roger Maris's long-standing record for home runs hit in a single season. Both broke Maris's record, but McGwire ultimately came out on top, hitting a record seventy home runs that year.

In the now more than a decade since the home run race, however, there has been growing speculation that one or both players may have surpassed Maris's record with the help of ana-bolic steroids or other performance-enhancing drugs. Both play-ers, who had been solid but not exceptional sluggers in the past, suddenly exhibited a spike in home runs, although both denied using steroids. Most damaging to McGwire was his former team-mate José Canseco's allegations that McGwire had used performance-enhancing drugs for years before breaking the record. When subpoenaed to testify in front of a congressional committee, McGwire refused to speak about his alleged steroid use under oath, leaving fans and sportswriters alike to draw their own conclusions about his innocence or guilt.

Mark McGwire's eligibility for baseball's Hall of Fame began during the 2006–2007 season. Many baseball writers, such as Ann Killion of the San Jose Mercury News, *had qualms about voting for a player with such a blemish on his record. In the fol-lowing viewpoint Killion describes her reasons for withholding her vote for McGwire, citing not only the published criteria for Hall of Fame inclusion but also her own ethical misgivings. Ap-*

Ann Killion, "Killion: Why McGwire Won't Be Getting My Hall Vote," *San Jose Mercury News*, December 19, 2006. Copyright © 2006, San Jose Mercury News, Calif. Repro-duced by permission.

parently many other sportswriters shared Killion's reluctance, because McGwire received less than one-quarter of the votes needed on that initial ballot.

Killion is an award-winning sports columnist who writes for the San Jose Mercury News *and* Sports Illustrated. *She is one of the longest-tenured female sports writers in the country, having covered seven Olympic Games, five World Cups, and many other significant sporting events.*

I finally plucked my responsibility out of the pile of other December demands—wish lists, unlabeled envelopes, menu plans.

It's my Baseball Writers' Association 2007 Hall of Fame ballot. And this year it's a daunting duty. Bigger than Christmas dinner for 23.

It's the inaugural juice ballot. The names on the list include Ken Caminiti, Jose Canseco and Mark McGwire. As a voter, I'm entrusted to help pass judgment on the steroid era's lasting legacy.

And here's how I'll determine my vote: Can I look my kids in the eyes when I tell them whom I selected?

I have no problem telling them the names I checked Monday. Two I've already voted for: Andre Dawson and Goose Gossage. And I'm voting for two first-timers: Tony Gwynn and Cal Ripken Jr.

I'm not voting for McGwire. What would I tell my kids, who saw my disgust at the congressional hearings in March 2005 and have heard my opinion over the years? "Sure, I think he cheated, but look at the rate at which he hit homers! Let's enshrine him forever!"

Some will say I'm playing God by withholding my vote. That I'm being the morality police. But that's actually what the Hall of Fame asks me to be. Voters are requested to factor in moral conclusions.

Here is rule No. 5: "Voting shall be based upon the player's record, playing ability, integrity, sportsmanship, character and contributions to the team(s) on which the player played."

Integrity, sportsmanship and character. Those are the judgments that I'm being asked to make.

I wasn't going to vote for McGwire before the congressional hearings, though they were a beautiful display of a lack of integrity and character, one that only makes my vote that much easier.

I watched McGwire morph over the years into a one-dimensional cartoon player, hearing the whispers the entire way. I took note when andro was found in his locker. I've read Canseco's accusations. I've absorbed the confessional testimony of his protege, Jason Giambi. I think McGwire's Hall of Fame credentials are based only on his home-run numbers, which I believe were inflated by performance-enhancing drugs.

So I'm not voting for him. And I don't buy the arguments I've heard put forth by the pro-McGwire voters. Such as:

1. If I don't vote for McGwire, how can I vote for anyone else from the steroid era?

Here's how: Go by your gut. The baseball voters I respect the most concede that their determinations are based primarily on a gut instinct. When they watched the guy, they knew at the end of the day—statistics aside—whether they were watching a Hall of Famer. Use the same criteria when considering steroids. Imperfect perhaps, but that's baseball.

2. Even if he was using steroids, it wasn't against the rules of baseball.

All the more reason to factor in steroids in the Hall of Fame vote. Steroids were illegal by law without a prescription. We know why baseball turned a blind eye—for fear of alienating sponsors and fans and seeing profits drop. All the more reason that voters, who have no vested financial interest in protecting the reputation of the game, should consider the illegitimate impact of steroids.

3. Even if he used steroids, McGwire captivated the nation in 1998 and saved baseball. That moment can never be taken away.

Then go back into the Hall of Fame balloting and elect Roger Maris. Because without Maris' single-season home run record—without that feat—McGwire could never have had his spine-tingly moment that made grown baseball writers cry. But Maris isn't in the Hall of Fame.

4. Whatever happened to innocent until proven guilty?

This isn't a court of law. And even if it was, all of the evidence in the steroid case isn't in. There might be late-in-life confessions. There might be apologies. There might even be a change of heart, by voters like me.

But it's not a legal situation. It's not a ballplayer's right—hit so many home runs and you're automatically enshrined. It is an honor and it is forever.

5. The Hall of Fame is full of cheaters and bums.

Maybe so, but I didn't vote for them. And all I can do is cast my own vote judiciously. And be able to look my kids in the eyes when I do it.

The Costs of Steroid Use

Men's Health

In the following viewpoint, a steroid user discusses his experiences with multiple steroid cycles. The author believed that he needed the aid of steroids in order to achieve his dream physique. While he claims he is close to the body he has always wanted, it came at a cost—both financially and physically.

Men's Health is a men's magazine that covers fitness, sexuality, nutrition and other aspects of men's lives.

At the end of 1996, I had been training hard for 12 years, and the results were obvious. At 5-foot-8, I had built myself up from 95 pounds to a high of 230, though 210 was about the most I could carry without looking chubby. I had 17-inch arms and was one of the strongest guys at my gym, squatting more than 500 pounds and pressing 140-pound dumbbells overhead. I had done very well in several drug-tested bodybuilding shows and had been featured in magazines.

But I was still nowhere near the physique I had dreamed of since high school. I wanted more size and better shape, and achieving this goal naturally seemed impossible.

You Use, You Lose

I began my first steroid cycle 6 years ago, when I was 27 years old. My wife was upset, but I had researched the subject, and convinced her I wasn't risking my health. Within a few weeks I gained nearly 20 pounds, and every single lift went up 20 to 30 percent. My muscles had a fuller look, as if inflated with air or pumped full of water. I felt I could work out for hours if I wanted.

My sex drive also went through the roof, and my wife complained about my increasing demands. Other, more negative side effects included water retention in my face and disgusting, boil-like acne pustules across my back and shoulders. But the worst impact was on my reputation at the gym. I'd been a vocal opponent of steroid use for the 4 years I'd trained there, and now I was Mr. Hypocrite.

I lost a few good friends.

Now, 6 years and about 12 cycles later, I weigh a solid 240 pounds, although I diet down to 210 when I enter bodybuilding competitions. My arms are up to 19 inches, and, although injuries have kept my strength from improving dramatically, I'm finally close to the look I always wanted.

That muscle came at a price. I've spent close to $30,000 on steroids and now stay on them at least two-thirds of the year. I have masses of scar tissue in my glutes from hundreds of injections. People I meet are intimidated, and some automatically assume I'm a jerk, which I'm not. But that's all trivial compared with this: A few months ago, after a cycle in which I had used a lot of oral steroids to prepare for a contest, a blood test showed liver damage comparable to that of a hepatitis patient.

Ruining Relationships

My liver has almost fully recovered, but now my wife wants me to quit. She says that at some stage I have to give up the idea of getting bigger and focus on my health, and I don't disagree. It's also getting harder to conceal my steroid use from the older of our two children.

Here's my advice to anyone considering steroids: Unless you're at or very near your maximum genetic potential, don't waste your time. Using steroids too soon will keep you from learning how to make gains without them. If you're under 23, you have no business juicing. Besides the fact you have enough natural testosterone, you could stunt your growth if you haven't reached your full adult height. Finally, most guys who set out to do "just one cycle" end up using steroids for years.

If you think you'll be the exception, you've just joined a very big club. Once you've started, it's tough to go back.

It's a personal choice, but one you have to think through as carefully as any other decision you make in life. Be sure you aren't going to let the desire to be huge take precedence.

A Casual Steroid User

Stephen Hirst

Stephen Hirst, the author of the following essay, was a skinny guy in college. His best friends, however, were always on steroids, and they had the bodies—and girlfriends—to prove it. On a dare, Hirst decided to do one cycle of the steroid Dianabol. In this essay, he recounts his fifty days on the drug, an experience that, he freely admits, had both positive and negative effects on his life.

Hirst readily acknowledges that he felt a little out of control while on steroids but says that he sometimes enjoyed the change from his usual mild-mannered ways. He also relished the grow- ing attention he received from both men and women for his body, something that was novel in his experience. Most of Hirst's negative response to the drugs, in fact, came when he stopped taking them. At that point, he started to understand just how great a toll the drugs were taking on his whole body, including both his physical and mental health. In the end, he reflects ironi- cally that his attempts to become hypermasculine ultimately left him feeling more emotional—more stereotypically feminine— than ever before.

Hirst obtained his MFA in writing from Eastern Washington University in Spokane, where he wrote for the Spokesman Re- view *newspaper. He currently lives in Brooklyn, New York, and works in Manhattan. This was his first published essay.*

Inside the Pi Kappa Alpha house I rapped my knuckles on a door at the end of a dark hallway. No one answered, but it was unlocked, and I stepped inside.

A pit-bull was tied to the bed, a long rope on its collar to give it the run of the room. She stared at me with wary black eyes but did not growl. This had to be Sammy.

Stephen Hirst, "A Casual Steroid User," *The Antioch Review*, vol. 66, Spring 2008, pp. 239–53. Copyright © 2008 by the Antioch Review, Inc. Reproduced by permission of the editors.

I waded in and began chatting with the animal.

"Howdy, girl . . . hey, now . . . don't maul Steve, now . . ."

She was calm, used to a steady stream of visitors. I scanned the room and spotted the microwave. The door swung open, the soft orange glow of the interior bulb the only light in the dark room. A plastic Ziploc bag sat in the center of the microwave with a yellow post-it note.

Steve, here is the D-ball. DO NOT TAKE MORE THAN ONE A DAY, and remember, DO NOT DRINK. Enjoy! Love, Zack

Looking Back

Six weeks earlier I sat with Zack in our friend T.J.'s apartment. Zack had broken it off with his girlfriend—in epic, disastrous fashion—a month or so earlier, and a chance encounter with her had set him off again. She had cheated on him—with two guys—at the same time—in a hot tub. He wasn't a sobbing emotional wreck or anything, just angry. He kept bouncing a tennis ball off the wall and catching it, sipping an Icehouse . [beer]. Zack was engaging in the time-honored tradition of getting over a break-up by aiming generalizations at the entire gender.

"You're looking at a whole new Zack, boys. The only bitch I care about from now on is tied up at the Pike [short for Pi Kappa Alpha] House in my room, eating kibble."

T.J. was sitting on the couch flipping channels. We were killing time before heading downtown. Restless, I went to the metal bar bolted to T.J.'s wall and began doing pull-ups.

"Look at scarecrow, flexing it," T.J. cracked. Both guys outweighed me by about sixty pounds. Zack took a long pull on his beer and watched as I started to tire. T.J. kept up the heckling. "Trying to do some pull-ups, skinny?"

"Shut it . . . dick-tree," I wheezed out between reps.

Zack spoke up in my defense. "He can probably do more than you."

"Yeah, well, I'm fat now, though. I haven't been lifting lately," T.J. said. I strained for one more repetition and almost didn't make it. "Hey, look at that!" T.J. yelled and bolted up from the couch, pointing out the "striations" in my shoulders. I nodded and pretended I knew what a "striation" was while the guys started to brainstorm.

"Can you imagine him on Deca [Deca-Durabolin, a steroid]?"

"What he needs to do is stack. Dianabol or Winstrol is what I would start him on." . . .

"So you guys think it would affect me differently?" I asked.

Zack launched into an animated lecture. "Oh, it would, man, it would. Deca hits skinny guys like a freight train. You'll see results in two, three days. It has to do with the faster metabolism."

I told them to forget it. Not going to happen. Steve Hirst draws a line at needle drugs. So we went downtown to help Zack forget about his ex, but I thought about what they said all night.

Summing Up What I Know

Sometime the next week I began to consider everything I knew and had read about steroids. They shrink your testicles. They cause acne. Involuntary rage. Mood swings. Reduced sperm count. Baldness. Increased risk of prostate cancer. When use is discontinued, testosterone production is halted for a time, so feminization may occur in men. Breasts can develop. In women, side effects can be deepening of the voice, facial hair, an enlarged clitoris, and thick, bony brows that can become permanent. Steroids can subtract years from your life span. Could it possibly be worth all that? Or were these warnings a bunch of worst-case-scenario scare tactics?

I'm six feet tall, weighed around 160 pounds in college, and was largely content with my build. That being said, I still wanted to sample the body of a 185-pound mini-hulk; try it on, take it around the block a few times. My days as an athlete were behind me, but I still wanted to know how it would feel to be stronger and faster than I'd ever been before.

I considered it like taking a test drive in a sports car that could be a lot of fun, but you know you're never going to buy. It may be hard to fathom the motivation involved, but—if women with an A or B cup size had an opportunity to go up to a *big* C or D for only eight weeks, without surgery, then return to the same body they knew, how many women would seize that chance? Considering the rising number of American women each year who opt to go under a knife for cosmetic reasons, I think it's safe to assume there'd be a large market for a product like that. The free drinks alone would make it at least a worthwhile experiment.

So I made my decision to lease a new type of body, with an option to buy.

My Conditions

Zack's cell rang twice before he picked up and I didn't wait for him to answer before laying out my conditions.

"Look, here's what I want. I don't want to inject anything, I don't want my back and face to break out like I'm fifteen, I don't want man-boobs, and I don't want my nuts to shrink."

Zack was quiet a moment. "Then you should get a tub of protein powder and stop bothering me, dick-mouth."

"Isn't there some kind of middle ground?" I pleaded.

"Are you worried about injecting? Listen, I can shoot you up. I didn't learn how to give myself the shots until my third cycle. My big brother got tired of looking at my ass. I'll show you how."

"Uh, thanks I guess, but that's not even the issue. Isn't there anything I can take with minimal side effects?"

He let out an exasperated breath. "I guess you can take *only* Dianabol, but you should really consider stacking."

Stacking?

Zack explained I should be combining two complementary steroids at once. In bodybuilding circles it is considered a bit of a waste to do only one and not the other—you're drinking the beer, so why not have a smoke, too? He sounded dejected that I didn't want to go all-out and stack, but he could have fifty pills—one cycle—available in two weeks.

"Forget everything you've heard," he said. "Your boys may tighten or even shrink a little, but they always bounce back." With Dianabol alone (D-ball for short), I wouldn't have to worry about that, or acne, too much. As for the "roid rage," Zack warned that a lot of people did become overly defensive, and that if a fight ever broke out I would likely find myself the first to dive into the fray. Some users crave confrontation. I was also to expect an increase in sex drive.

According to Zack, the man-mammaries were a rare nightmare scenario. That only happened to *career* juice-balls, guys who used in cycles for years, gained tons of muscle, and then stopped lifting and quit cold-turkey. And one more thing: "You feel awesome," Zack said in a faraway voice. "You wake up earlier, you feel like sprinting up the side of a mountain, you feel like howling at the f--king *moon*, dog. You have to understand, this is a *fun* drug. It's a real rush."

So I settled on just the D-ball. I'd managed to rationalize the risks to myself with Zack's help, but I still knew his frat boy pseudo-science couldn't be taken as airtight. He was a good friend, but now that he was my drug dealer and I was a customer, he was going to hype his product.

The New Steroid User

The assumption is that steroids are only for athletes and bodybuilders, but that's a limited segment of the user base, and an outdated stereotype. The new steroid user is more likely to be using not to enhance athletic performance, but to look better at the beach. It's big with entertainers—Hollywood and the music industry, all those whose line of work involves displaying their bodies. A lot of users just enjoy how the juice makes them feel, both physically and psychologically. For some it becomes almost recreational, the "fun drug."

And then, some are more interested in results other than looking buff. Police are a quickly growing part of this market. They crave the physical edge steroids provide, plus the boost in confidence and aggression that accompanies the testosterone increase.

For some, the temptation to supplement income by dealing at the local gym becomes irresistible. It's a growing problem that's still very much under the radar when steroids are discussed. People are quick to condemn pro athletes, but few realize the danger of encountering an officer answering a call of "shots fired" with testosterone levels fifty times higher than normal. As early as 1991, the *FBI Law Enforcement Bulletin* ran a piece stating that "anabolic steroid abuse by police officers is a serious problem that merits greater awareness by departments across the country."

However, the users I'm best acquainted with are the frat boys. At the University of Central Florida in 2002, steroid use was fairly rampant. The Pikes were notorious for this, being veined and muscle-bound, with hair-trigger tempers. Other fraternities had their share of users, but the Pikes presented a united front of artificial testosterone. I once asked Zack how many of his [frat] brothers were juicing at any given time.

"Jesus, everybody," he said, shrugging his shoulders. "Basically everybody who lives in the house, at some point has been on the juice. I guess there are maybe six or seven guys who don't mess with it at all."

The Pikes had a hideous reputation on campus. Many women viewed them as a sort of primitive, subhuman/ Morlock[1]creature. While on the surface this didn't seem to matter—there were always plenty of beautiful, willing women

1. Morlocks are subhuman, physically strong creatures who live underground in H.G. Wells's futuristic novel *The Time Machine*.

at the Pike House—there were also a fair number of women who vowed never to set foot inside the place. There were always shady stories floating around school, whispers of a punch spiked with GHB [gamma-hydroxybutyric acid, a so-called date-rape drug] at an off-campus party, or sightings of Pikes carrying women out of a club over their shoulders like sacks of grain and loading them into cars.

Zack was aware of these rumors, and angrily denounced them as jealous rumbling. But they weren't exactly a friendly bunch—many students, even other frat boys, referred to them as the "Asshole Frat," and they did little to erase this image. It wasn't an arduous stretch to think that some of the stories held a little bit of truth; maybe a lot.

Getting Ready

For the two weeks before I began my cycle, I prepared as instructed. I bought an economy size bottle of [the herb] milk thistle, a supplement for liver health. Steroids can damage the liver, and combining alcohol can tax it beyond tolerance. I loaded up my fridge with lunch meats and other protein-packed foods. Chicken and ground beef took over my freezer, sliced turkey and ham packed the crisper, banana clusters lurked in every corner of the kitchen. In the morning I mixed protein powder into my milk. Constant eating is encouraged. Hunger can make a juicer extra irritable, so you never want to be without some protein bars or a bag of beef jerky.

With D-ball the body seems to harvest protein more effectively than it was ever intended to. It's not unheard of for users in their first three or four days to wake up with *visibly* more muscle mass than they went to bed with.

The first morning after I got back from the Pike House I took one itty-bitty round dull-orange pill, smaller than an aspirin. I ate a breakfast of scrambled eggs, sausage, Cookie Crisps, and pink grapefruit before meeting T.J. at the gym where he worked. I was the smallest guy in the room by forty or fifty pounds. His gym looked like the set of a professional wrestling tryout. There were juicers lifting and grunting everywhere. We ran through an hour and a half session, T.J. teaching me some new lifting exercises along the way. My favorite was what he called the "Hulk Flex" exercise, named for a [famed professional wrestler-turned-actor] Hulk Hogan trademark show-off move. Pulleys connected to the weight stack were held out to the side at chest level. I watched as T.J. began his motion there and pulled his arms down into a position at his waist, fists pointed down and shaking with tension, holding the pose for a few seconds. When it was my turn my entire body shook with the strain of stabilizing the stack.

That day didn't feel much different from a regular workout. I had been lifting weights on and off since sophomore year of high school, when I'd decided to stop being a skinny punk and become a slightly more chiseled skinny punk. I could always achieve good definition, but it's hard for thin guys to pack on muscle. Our metabolisms are determined to burn everything up before that can happen. That night, I drank a protein shake and went to sleep, but first I paused in front of the mirror. I gazed at my triceps, rotating my arm from side to side, and tried to picture how it would look when the juice kicked in. I smirked at the skinny guy and said goodbye to that schmuck—for the next fifty days. . . .

Results

The next morning I still felt like me. I was beginning to wonder about the quality of Zack's connection, but then I noted I was hardly even sore for having just lifted so intensely—even after months of relative inactivity. The lack of soreness meant it was working. I gave the weights a day off and did floor exercises, pushups, crunches. At work I ordered the half-chicken (instead of the quarter-chicken) and potatoes with green beans for lunch. My second symptom—an up-tick in appetite.

By the third day something had definitely changed. I was awake at seven in the morning, and I usually slept until around nine. I woke up hungry, tromped downstairs, and began sizzling bacon while munching a bowl of Cookie Crisps with slices of bananas.

After work, I stopped in at the gym for an evening session. I looked at myself in the mirror behind the dumbbell rack and froze. My bicep was rigid and tight, puffed up as if I was curling a weight at that very moment—and I wasn't even flexing. Even though I hadn't lifted since Monday, I retained the post workout "pump" that usually recedes after an hour or so. It stayed with me all that night.

Soon, I did notice an increase in the attention I was getting from the girls. Mostly more flirting, more glances and eye contact when I was out, particularly at my weekend job lifeguarding at the Y. It's possible I was just more attuned to it, paying better attention to who was looking.

I admit I had been most curious about the reaction from women, even psyched, but it was mainly dudes who noticed, other gym rats.

"Hirst, you're huge, man! You're like the incredible hulk—my boy's been in the gym," Mike said to me at a party. I had been there all night and no one had really noticed my inflated look except another *guy*. It's a lot like the way only women notice what shoes the others are wearing, or some subtle cosmetic tweak. This was a little disappointing. Looking back, I question my motives—was I trying to satisfy a curiosity, or was I trying to mimic Zack, thinking of the hordes of leggy foxes who were always begging for a piece of him? Both, but I think it may have been more of the latter than I was willing to admit to myself at the time. A part of me then reasoned that if I assumed the trappings of Zack (minus the metro shirts and hair gel, I mean) it couldn't hurt my cause.

Day seven and I was overflowing with energy. I ate a Meat Lover's Skillet at Denny's to start my morning, and drove to work scarfing a pack of peanuts. A humming undercurrent of explosive power sang through my veins, shrieking to be channeled and used. The thought of sitting in my cubicle was killing me. I rolled down the window and gulped in the outside air. Sunlight poured through the open window, heating the left side of my body, fueling me. As the rays beat down, I drew power from this energy source. It felt like I'd become a sort of solar battery, and I conversed with the yellow giant.

"Mmm . . . sun. How I love you, sun. Bless and warm me with your harmful ultraviolet rays, and I shall receive your divine radiation with a glad heart."

The hands on the clock at work seemed to struggle through a mass of peanut butter. I stretched my coffee breaks to the limit. My lunch of a turkey sandwich with a protein bar and apple juice seemed a pittance. I flew to the gym from the office and hit the free weights, driven.

First I did three sets of incline bench, then decline. After squats and some leg press, I realized my chest wasn't very tired or sore, so I went back to working it with the flat bench, and threw in some rowing. I stayed for nearly two and a half hours. It was becoming much easier to motivate myself to get up and go to the gym, partly because I was seeing new strength gains every day—instant results! The impossible promise of American marketing, delivered!

"A Second Puberty"

On the day of my fourteenth dosage I strutted into the mall, thrumming with the testosterone levels of a lowland silverback gorilla. Passing through the food court, a petite Hispanic woman in a little slip of an orange top caught my attention. At first my eye was attracted by the vivid orange, but then I was studying the tight fabric stretched across her chest, deep-set black eyes, and the slope of her neck where it met shoulder.

She caught me staring and I hastened along, but the biology was kicking in. Moments later she was forgotten, a single lost page in a flip-book of women that I unfailingly eye-f--ked with abandon as they roamed the mall. I was indiscriminate and blatant, checking out moms, sorority girls, emo girls, Goth girls, the chick behind the counter at Orange Julius, the shoe department woman at JC Penney. I caught a pair of tanned soccer legs walking away from me out of the corner of my eye, and admired them until I noticed their owner's jacket said "Winter Park HS Soccer," and that's when I bolted out of there.

Any ideas of my having a "type" flew out the window. It was like middle school all over again, a second puberty. I desired *woman* now with a laser-beam focus that would let me think of little else unless I sublimated all of it into a two-and-a-half-hour session at the gym. Around day thirty I was one seventy-two, twelve pounds heavier than when I'd started. The most noticeable gains were in my shoulders, but my arms had also been transformed into corded, veined spectacles.

Road Rage

One morning I was up early, [driving] . . . to get a friend at the airport before work, when a white Neon pulled up next to me at a light.

"Hey, asshole," a voice said. I turned. In the driver's seat sat a "Johnny Badass" character in a wife beater and a Dolphins hat.

"Excuse me?"

"You heard me. You cut me off and almost made us wreck back there."

"Well, I didn't even see you, partner. Sorry if I did, but—"

"Fine, then this time you get out of an ass-kicking," he said, and this kindled something. His arrogance seeded a desire in me to hurl something. *I'm just trying to be nice about the situation, and this ass-hat thinks I'm afraid? Well, piss on you, Jack.* A coppery taste rose up in my mouth and my neck heated. I didn't think, but instinctively scrabbled for something heavy on the seat, the floor, anywhere. When my hand found something I whipped it through my passenger window at Johnny Badass's face. Turned out it was a mostly full glass bottle of Arizona iced tea, which thunked solidly off the top of his door and fell inside the window, but didn't break. The driver yelped in shock. Words were exchanged, we each shouted some threats, but surprise, he didn't want to leave the car anymore. I was angrier and louder than he was, and he couldn't match (or fake) the purity of the rage I was bringing to the table. I puttered along slowly with the prick staying several cars behind, and I remember how it felt, *loving* the knowledge that he was purposely going slower to avoid the awkward stoplight reunion with the crazy guy. I'm not the most serene driver *off* juice. On it, I became a doubly enraged unmanageable monster, a condition I've dubbed "Road-Roid Rage." All that day at work I was angry, snapping at undeserving coworkers.

That night I paused in front of the mirror as I exited the shower. I spun around and studied myself from all angles, finding back muscles and lines of definition I hadn't known existed. My triceps jutted from my upper arms so far that all my sleeves were becoming tight. I arched my back and "drew the bow" in the Apollo pose, chuckling. It was hard to believe I had transformed myself so much in so little time.

Withdrawal

Forty-five days into my cycle I got the flu. I took the last five pills as scheduled, even though I couldn't drag myself into the gym. I half-heartedly did floor exercises, but the sickness sapped my vigor, and it took me about a week to fully recover. I got lazy, tired of lifting all the time. It was getting boring. I made the rookie user's mistake of going cold turkey and not working out for over a week. As I learned later, it is much better to taper off this stuff. There are even drugs you can take to lessen side effects of the comedown. Side effects like depression and feminization.

All at once testosterone is ratcheting back down and estrogen is shooting up. Stopping in the middle of such leaping gains is like slamming on the brakes of a speeding locomotive. It takes a toll on the whole structure.

Finally I made it into the gym one afternoon for a quick lift after work. My strength had ebbed already. I was forced to lower the weight on each station, often more than once, and it was depressing. I left after only an hour and there was a message on my phone from Zack. He said something about forgetting to tell me I should stop by and pick up something called Clomid, to even out my system when I quit. I soon forgot about this message. I was starting a new job in a couple of days, and didn't think about it again.

The next few weeks were bad. I was sluggish at work, taking forever to complete even brainless mail-room tasks. My mood was all over the place. I hated everybody and they all became stupid and annoying.

The most glaring physical withdrawal symptom was the expected one: I got smaller. At the peak of my usage I was 179 pounds. In a few weeks my weight was down to 166. I retreated indoors and glued myself to the couch in a funk. There were still moments when a desire gripped me, insisting I rattle out crunches and push-ups, but I seldom had the energy or willpower to follow through. I was always tired after work and went straight home. *I'm deteriorating*, I thought, *every day I don't go to the gym I lose more ground*. I could feel my body losing hardness, becoming mushier, less efficient. I didn't lift or run because I was tired, and didn't have any energy because I wasn't running and lifting.

For weeks after I quit, my emotions pin-balled all over, but mostly downward. I felt stressed about some unknown but imminent calamity, always under pressure. The body does not resume producing testosterone right away. Once you've been getting your testosterone from a pill for a while, your testicles decide they can take a little vacation from producing it. Driving on the interstate or a busy downtown street, I would scream at perceived road offenses with my windows up, often shouting so loudly that people outside the car heard me. Once or twice I even teared up for no discernible reason before going in to work in the morning, just from thinking about too many things at once, or at a sentimental life-insurance commercial. Friends were concerned, people kept asking if I needed to talk. I hadn't told many people about my experiment, so only a few suspected what I was dealing with.

My testicles kicked back into production when I was at my lowest ebb, and my head began to sort itself out. I gave myself a stern lecture/pep-talk in the mirror. *Of course it will get better. It isn't that bad NOW, you idiot. Stop being so dramatic. Stop your bitching. Stop being so f--king WEAK.* I just kept telling myself that things would improve, that I couldn't keep feeling this crazy forever, and finally I didn't.

Lessons Learned

My curiosity about steroids had been satisfied, and I was still living down the effects of a so-called lightweight one. However, my testicles made it through intact and un-shrunk, the dreaded man-boobs never came near, and though the roids kicked my ass a little at the end, I can't say I regret the experience.

That body was bigger, faster, and ballsier than what I was used to driving. When you've been tooling around forever in a four-cylinder Civic and you rent a V8 Mustang, it's tough to go back. I remain fascinated by the fact that I felt—and looked—so vital and healthy on the Dianabol, yet all the while it was playing hell with my insides, putting a strain on my organs as well as doing a number on my psyche. I was ready to embrace the positive cosmetic changes and weather the bad ones, but it was the emotional changes that caught me off guard. I've always felt, rather arrogantly and naively considering my family's history of depression, that I can *will* myself out of low points. But when I went off the juice it was another story; there was a persistent gloominess that was harder to shake. It took time and effort.

I also gained a glimpse into how it would feel to be a T.J. or a Zack. Usually, I'm a friendly, accessible person. But when I was juicing there was an edge to my personality that is usually present only when I'm in a very dark mood. I noticed people treating me differently. A lot of people, especially those who hadn't known me long or my more academic friends, were especially deferential and jumpy, as if at any moment I might leap across the room and shatter jawbones. This deference made me a little uncomfortable, but at the same time I *liked* it.

I'd expected the hyper-masculine side effects—it was the post-dosage withdrawal period and the feminine side effects I hadn't anticipated.

"Sounds to me like you were on the rag," a female friend of mine offered. "The crying jags, the moodiness and depression . . . you were having PMS," she said, stifling laughter. Another woman, a neighbor of mine, agreed.

"It's a rare gift. Now you understand how we feel five days out of every month."

The irony wasn't lost on me; my quest to achieve a heightened sense of maleness ended with the opposite effect. In my rush to get huge I ended up having to deal with an emotional maelstrom akin to PMS, and became more like a chick than ever, cursed like Tiresias [in Greek mythology, Tiresias was transformed into a woman for seven years]. The plummet from gorilla-man to girly-man was sudden and stressful, and I wish it on nobody. Although I must admit to appreciating the sheer value of the two-for-one experience, and I guess I'm more sympathetic now, not as quick to dismiss women's complaints during that time of the month. I gleefully accepted changes like the angry outbursts and the supercharged sex drive, but the horrific glimpse inside PMS is something I never want to deal with again—and I didn't have to contend with bloating or cramps. Maybe Tiresias didn't have to either, or he might have felt differently.

So people were scared of me, and it was a power trip to be intimidating for a change, but it's good I bailed when I did. I like my hair, and would like to keep it for at least a while longer. I like my testicles the size they are. I like my liver. And, I like myself—far more now than I did at age twenty-one.

But it was a far from negative experience. You do miss things about it. Not as much the basking in the gloriousness of your own David-esque [after Michelangelo's sculpture] appearance, or the swiveling heads of moms bringing their kids in for swim class at the Y. Mainly you miss the feeling of something extra animating things inside, propelling you along toward whatever new reckless impulse seizes you, making you "desirous of everything at once." Or to use Zack's words— "you feel like howling at the f--king *moon*, dog. . . ."

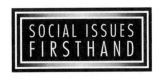

CHAPTER 2

Regulating Performance-Enhancing Drugs

Just Don't Get Caught

Patrik Sinkewitz, interviewed by Udo Ludwig and Detlef Hacke

Patrik Sinkewitz is a professional cyclist from Germany. During the 2007 Tour de France, he suffered a serious crash, colliding with a spectator during a mountainous descent in the Alps. While Sinkewitz was hospitalized, awaiting surgery for his injuries, it was revealed that he had tested positive for testosterone during a pre-Tour training camp in the Pyrenees Mountains.

During the investigation that followed, Sinkewitz cooperated with officials, speaking out not only about his own history of doping but also about the prevalence of doping practices on a team of which he was a member from 2003 to 2005. In exchange for his testimony, he was given only a one-year suspension from the sport and was able to return to professional cycling in July 2008.

In the following interview with the German magazine Der Spiegel, *Sinkewitz takes a matter-of-fact attitude toward doping, acknowledging its prevalence and freely admitting that the use of banned substances and procedures were customary aspects of many cyclists' routine. He explains some of the methods used to evade testing and to maximize performance. The interview took place during his suspension from the sport, and Sinkewitz expresses his desire to return to professional cycling, saying, "I don't know how to do anything else."*

After his suspension was lifted in 2008, Sinkewitz competed in the 2009 Tour of Portugal.

*D*er Spiegel: Mr. Sinkewitz, how did you find out about the positive results of your doping test?

Sinkewitz: It was around noon on July 18, [2007,] three days after my accident. I had been given a sedative and was being taken to the operating room in a wheelchair. My phone rang, but I didn't recognize the number.

Who was it?

I don't remember, perhaps a journalist. He asked me to comment on the fact that I had tested positive for testosterone in a random test at a training session on June 8. June 8? Testosterone? I really didn't understand what he was talking about. I told him that I was about to go into surgery. I remember that I was wondering where I could get more information. But I was under anesthesia 10 minutes later.

When you received the call, was it already clear to you that you had been caught?

No, I wasn't fully aware of it until the next morning. The patient in the bed next to me told me that the newspapers were reporting on the test, and it was on television all day long. I stayed in Hamburg a few more days, and during that time I received a visit from Rolf Aldag, the sporting director at T-Mobile [Sinkewitz's sponsor]. He advised me to tell the truth.

Telling the Truth

And what is it? What exactly happened in the Pyrenees?

The whole thing was bizarre. I had two or three small, 25 mg bags of testosterone gel in my wallet.

You just happened to have the stuff on you?

Yes.

Hard to believe.

But that's the way it was. I can't explain it either. I rubbed the contents of one bag onto my upper arm on the evening of June 7, just before I went to bed. I thought: Well, it can't hurt. I flushed the packaging down the toilet.

You hadn't been doing too well before that, and the Tour, the most important race of the season, was fast approaching. Was that why you resorted to the drug?

I was concerned about my form, despite the victory at the Frankfurt Grand Prix. The year hadn't gone the way I had expected, especially at the classic races. After you've lost a couple of races, you start to wonder whether the others are faster than you because they're getting a little extra boost. The crazy thing is that I really wasn't under any pressure. My contract wasn't going to expire until the end of 2008, and everyone was satisfied with me. But I wasn't. I always wanted to improve.

How did the doping test happen the next day?

Five of us went on a long ride, more than 200 kilometers (124 miles). We got back to the hotel at about 8 p.m. We knew that inspectors were there waiting for us. A masseur had notified our sporting director. It was normal for us to be tested at the training camp.

Just Part of the Routine

Testosterone is easy to detect. Weren't you in a panic?

Not at all. I wasn't in the least bit concerned after the test.

Why not? Don't you consider a small bag of testosterone doping?

I knew, of course, that it's prohibited. But I assumed the amount wouldn't be detectable. I also didn't feel that I had done anything wrong.

You knew that you had broken the rules, but you thought it was nothing?

That was our approach to it as cycling pros. I didn't think anything of it when I put the stuff on my arm. I'll probably never really know why I did it. I can count off on one hand the number of times I've used testosterone gel—because it doesn't really do much. But taking something to improve my performance just happened to be a part of my life.

"Just Don't Get Caught!"

T-Mobile introduced a strict anti-doping policy in 2007. You must have been aware of it. Or didn't the team management make that clear enough to you?

Of course they were saying: No doping! But as a rider, it's difficult to believe that things can really change from one day to the next. You're still expected to do well. The message I understood was this: Just don't get caught! But now I know that they were really serious about it.

What else did you take this year besides testosterone?

Cortisone.

That was it?

Yes. The risks were too great. T-Mobile had introduced internal tests. And besides, during training we could expect to see inspectors come knocking at our door at any time.

You became a professional cyclist at 20, and now you're 27. Is it possible that you've become addicted to performance-enhancing drugs?

I wouldn't call it an addiction. But the truth is, when you join a team as a new professional you encounter a system. As a young rider, older riders let you know how the business works. You're ambitious, you train hard, you develop professionally and, at some point, you give yourself that extra boost. Things just keep getting better, you're successful, you get recognition, everyone likes you and everyone loves you. That's how doping becomes normal.

Someone to Blame

When your case was revealed to the public, there were special broadcasts about it on television, and Germany's public TV stations cancelled their live reporting on the Tour de France. Rarely has a positive test set off such a furor.

I was the right rider at the right time, the one they could blame for everything. Suddenly it was all my fault: the anti-doping policy's lack of credibility, the TV networks' decision to cancel their coverage, and the notion that supposedly nothing has changed. I couldn't just sit back and watch. There were many people who also took advantage of my case to improve their own public images.

T-Mobile rider Linus Gerdemann said that he was "furious" with you, that you had jeopardized "our team and our approach." Other riders on the team reacted similarly. Do you understand your fellow cyclists' anger?

Riders called me up afterwards to say that they had had no other choice. I couldn't understand the way they changed their tune. I didn't harm anyone, nor did I cause anyone to lose his job. It's a great disappointment to me to hear someone with whom I've shared a room for weeks making those kinds of statements, especially because I wasn't in a position to defend myself. Sometimes it's a brutal profession. The first thing I thought of at the time was revenge. I have a more levelheaded take on the issue today.

Do you feel that you were treated unfairly?

I made a big mistake. There's no doubt about it. But there have been positive testing cases in the past where the offender wasn't attacked to quite the same extent, especially not by other riders.

Do you also feel unfairly treated because you know, or at least have an idea, that you're not the only one, and that others are still doping?

I'd rather not comment on that.

Under Investigation

Prosecutors in Bonn are now investigating you on suspicions that you deceived your contractual partners. Were you surprised by this investigation?

The truth is that things were already going so poorly for me that nothing surprised me anymore. But then the BKA [Bundeskriminalamt, Germany's version of the FBI] sent 20 agents to search my house. They even paid a visit to my parents and my ex-girlfriend. My mother had to justify the fact that she had heart pills. When she demanded an explanation, the agent, who even had a pistol in his belt, said to her: "I'm the one asking the questions here." I gave them a saliva sample that evening, and they also took my fingerprints. Okay, I screwed up, but the whole thing is exaggerated. I'm not a hardened criminal.

What did the officers find?

Ampoules containing cortisone, testosterone gel residues, syringes and needles, a centrifuge for measuring my blood values. And receipts for EPO [erythropoietin, a blood builder] from the spring of 2006. But, contrary to the erroneous reports in the press, they didn't find any EPO or growth hormone.

Reports that you had said that world champion Paolo Bettini gave you performance-enhancing drugs caused an uproar at the cycling world championship in Stuttgart in September. Was that what you said?

No. I was shopping when Bettini called me to tell me what I had supposedly accused him of. But the whole thing was a misunderstanding. It's possible that the name Bettini came up at some point during a conversation with the German Cycling Federation's anti-doping commission, but I certainly didn't claim that he gave me any drugs. They made that up. Bettini warned me: If you said that, then things could get dangerous for you.

Was doping part of the deal from the very beginning of your career?

No. I spent my first two years as a professional with Mapei in Italy, on their youth team. We rode in minor races. Doping wasn't an issue.

Mapei withdrew as a sponsor in late 2002. That was when you switched to Quick Step in Belgium and started riding in big races. How were things with your new team?

Different.

They quickly made it clear to you that doping was the thing to do?

Yes. The way it was framed was that everyone was doing it. As if it were part of being a professional. Everyone knew it, but no one wanted to admit it. You didn't talk about it.

"I'm Not the One Who Invented Doping"

How did you learn how to dope—from other riders, from doctors?

A little bit from everyone. After all, I'm not the one who invented doping.

Which drugs did you use?

At the time, and this certainly isn't a secret anymore, EPO was the drug of choice. Then there were things like cortisone and Synacthene [a "stealth drug" undetectable before 2009]. I didn't know anything about blood doping in those days.

EPO has been detectable since 2000. How did you manage to pass the tests?

When I found out that a dose is detectable for five days, I stopped using the drug six days before a race. There were hardly any random tests during training in those days.

Was Patrick Lefevere, the manager of Quick Step, aware of what was going on in his team?

It's hard to imagine that he couldn't have known. There are things you don't talk about, but they're still clear to everyone. I don't know the extent to which he was aware of the details.

Under Pressure

You were already being hailed as the new Jan Ullrich after your triumph at the 2004 Deutschland Tour. Were you just as euphoric as everyone else?

No. I didn't take it seriously when the media made such a big deal about me. Someone like Jan Ullrich only comes along once. I was never as good as he was. But it was clear to me that I had potential. I was only 23, and I had everything ahead of me. But the pressure was still mounting. A fourth-place finish wasn't anything special anymore.

Why did you decide to switch to T-Mobile in 2006?

It was a financially lucrative offer. Besides, they gave me a three-year contract, which was worth a lot in itself. It seemed to me that, as a German rider, being part of a German team was an option for a secure future.

Autotransfusion

Autotransfusion [transfusing an individual with blood previously removed, to increase the number of red blood cells] became a standard method in 2005. Did you do this at Quick Step?

No. I didn't find out what it is and how it works until the summer of 2005. T-Mobile was doing well in the big races, which led me to believe that they must have been doing it.

Andreas Schmid and Lothar Heinrich, both at the University of Freiburg Hospital, were the T-Mobile team doctors. Did you ask them about it?

I specifically asked them about it at our first meeting in November 2005. I was told that it was a possibility. But it was my impression that the Freiburg doctors didn't like doing it. In fact, they were really against it. But apparently they wanted to prevent riders from finding someone else to do it and risking that something could go wrong.

What makes you think that?

They never pressured me to do it. They never said that I had to do it. It was my idea.

Didn't you have any misgivings?

No. They were using my own blood—what could be risky about that? It seemed a lot safer to me than drugs. And it was very effective.

Did you consider it doping?

Riders don't use that word, anyway. Your main concern is not to get caught.

In blood doping, they draw about half a liter of your own blood and reinfuse it after about a month. Isn't this an unpleasant procedure?

As a pro, I'm already used to dealing with a few unpleasant things. But I can't imagine that a rider would voluntarily consent to blood doping.

Did you have to pay for the blood doping?

Only for the bags. It was maybe €50 [euros] apiece, I don't remember exactly how much.

Then who paid for it?

I have no idea. I assume that it didn't cost very much. I think they already had the necessary equipment and refrigerators there at the clinic.

Who at Team T-Mobile knew about the blood doping?

In theory, just the doctor and me.

You supposedly said, during questioning, that blood doping was systematic at Team T-Mobile beginning in 2006.

I didn't say that, because that's something I don't even know. It isn't like giving blood. We may have had an idea that other riders were receiving similar treatments, but no one knew exactly what the other guy was doing. In any event, I was always lying completely alone in the room on a cot.

Do you know whether you were the only one?

I don't want to comment on the other riders.

No Point to It Anymore

The apartments of Spanish doctor Eufemiano Fuentes were searched before the 2006 Tour de France. Ullrich was suspended, and so was T-Mobile's sporting director, Rudy Pevenage. Did you stop blood doping right away?

No. On the evening of the first stage, I drove from Strasbourg to Freiburg.

Ullrich, your fellow team member, had been suspended two days earlier for blood doping, and you actually had the nerve to continue using the same method?

Yes. The doctors really didn't want to do it anymore. But I said, look, we have the blood, so let's put it in. What was going to happen? It was already clear that it would be over after the Tour de France. Nobody wanted to take the risk anymore.

How were you prepared for the Tour?

I was actually supposed to get two bags. But there was something wrong with both of them. The blood just wouldn't flow. A little of the blood flowed from the first bag, but then it clotted, and the same thing happened with the second bag. So I basically rode the Tour without being doped. The doctor said that this had never happened. He was embarrassed. But I didn't ask for any further explanations. It wasn't something you asked about. It just made me angry. Tough luck, I thought.

Isn't it sort of unusual to get an entire liter of blood in one session?

The original plan was to administer the second bag 10 or 15 days later. But that would've meant making arrangements, and it had become too dangerous after the Ullrich affair. There was no way that the doctors were going to travel to France with the blood.

When did you give the blood?

I began giving the blood at the beginning of the year, so that we could build up a supply of two bags over time. You have to keep replacing the blood, because it goes bad after a month. I received a bag in April, but without giving any fresh blood. I was hoping that that would prepare me for the Classic. I went to Freiburg a total of four or five times for the same reason, and I was always at the clinic where normal examinations were also done.

At Schmid's and Heinrich's clinic.

I don't want to comment on that.

Dealing with Scandal

How did the team react when Ullrich was suddenly gone?

It was strange for us to have lost our captain. We thought it was unfair that he wasn't being allowed to ride, just because of some alleged evidence. Meanwhile, others who were supposedly on Fuentes's list were kept on the team. That was all we knew. At the time, there was no way of predicting everything else that would eventually happen.

Did you talk about the scandal with the team?

During the Tour, you're tense from morning to night. We talked about the stages on the bus ride to the hotel, not about doping. Of course, whenever was I asked in public whether I had doped, I always said no. It's part of my job.

When you stopped the blood doping after the Tour, were you concerned that it would hurt your performance?

I was relieved. There was no more stress. You have to realize that these things are increasingly stressful. Besides, I also know that I'm not a bad cyclist, even without doping.

The T-Mobile team received strict instructions after the Tour to stop doping. Did you come to terms with the fact that your performance would suffer at first?

Well, it was hard to imagine that everyone in other countries would play along with the anti-doping campaign. Everyone says: Of course we're against doping, but many don't really mean it. For example, I was hoping that I would be in the lead this year during the Paris-Nice stage. But then the Spaniards came along and cleaned up. It makes you wonder, after the race.

The Future of the Sport

Do you believe that the many confessions will be good for cycling?

Everyone told me to be honest and put my cards on the table. It hasn't helped me so far. I'm more than just somebody who sinned by doping. I'm the defendant in a crime. But telling the truth is also liberating. I don't have to hide anything anymore.

You're hoping for leniency. Why are you so determined to get back into cycling?

I don't know how to do anything else. Sometimes I think that there isn't any point to it anymore. Time is the only thing I have plenty of. I could find plenty of things to do, but when everything seems pointless, you end up doing nothing.

Are you in training?

I couldn't do anything at first, because of the injuries from my fall. I wanted to start up again after four or five weeks, but I couldn't do it. Now I'm back. I spent four hours riding through the woods on my mountain bike yesterday. I was totally exhausted. It was a great feeling.

Are you still in touch with some of your old fellow riders?

Almost all contacts ended from one day to the next. Some of the people I used to see almost every day contacted me once to see how I was doing. It was if I didn't even exist anymore. Before I tested positive, I had a three-year contract, a private sponsor and a house. And there were constantly people who were supporting me. Now I've lost my profession and I have nothing left but my house. I could use help now, but there's nobody left. Everyone knows that people pat you on the back when you're successful, but it comes as a shock to realize what it's like when the success is gone. It yanks the ground out from under your feet.

Are you ruined?

I don't make any money anymore, and I have to pay fines and lawyers. Besides, I didn't exactly make a fortune during my first few years as a professional. At least the house is paid off.

Under the terms of your contract with Team T-Mobile, you might have to pay back part of your salary.

I try not to think about that. It's something my attorney will deal with. I don't want to talk about it. Besides, what do they want from me? Haven't I been punished enough?

Prescription for Disaster

Gordon Bakoulis

Elite runner Gordon Bakoulis had accepted postrace urine testing as a fact of life; it was a minor inconvenience, but not a big deal since she had never done anything wrong. In 1992, however, she was shocked to be informed by the national track and field association that she had tested positive for a banned substance after a high-profile marathon. Bakoulis, who had been forced to take several weeks off from training earlier that year while she battled Lyme disease, had not known that one of the drugs prescribed for the disease was on the U.S. Olympic Committee's banned substance list. The drug was used by some athletes to block the presence of steroids in the body.

In this essay, Bakoulis acknowledges her own errors in judgment, admitting that as an elite athlete she was perhaps too naïve in her approach to prescription drugs. She also, however, points out the inherent unfairness in many of the established procedures for dealing with doping violations, arguing that an innocent mistake like hers should not be painted with the same broad brush as someone who is caught cheating.

Bakoulis was ultimately reinstated into USA Track & Field as a competitive runner and competed in the Olympic trials in 1996 and 2000. She is the author or editor of several books on running and cross training and has worked as an editor at Woman's Day, Running Times, *and* New York Runner *magazines. Her articles have appeared in a wide variety of health, fitness, women's interest, and parenting publications.*

On Wednesday, November 18, 1992, I received a phone call from Kathy Presnal, the substance abuse programs manager of The Athletics Congress (now USA Track & Field

Gordon Bakoulis, "Prescription for Disaster," *Runner's World*, vol. 28, October 1993, pp. 88–94. Copyright © 1993 Rodale, Inc. Reproduced by permission.

[USATF]). I wasn't alarmed by the call. I'd just spent a month in Colorado and hadn't yet told Kathy that I was back in New York City.

Nationally ranked runners—I've run a 2:33 marathon—are responsible for letting Kathy's office know where we are at all times. USATF tests athletes for drugs both in and out of competition. No matter where I am or what I'm doing, I can be asked to produce a urine sample within 48 hours. I assumed Kathy was phoning simply to check on my whereabouts.

I assumed wrong. Kathy was calling to tell me that I had tested positive for a banned substance at the New York City Marathon.

A Bad Dream?

"What was the substance?" I asked. I felt very calm. Obviously, this was either a bad dream or someone's idea of a joke.

"Probenecid," she answered. "It's a masking agent."

"I took that last summer for Lyme disease," I said. "What's a masking agent?" I still felt calm.

"It's a substance that hides the presence of other drugs, in this case by retaining them in the kidneys," she explained. "Did you call the USOC [United States Olympic Committee] Drug Hotline before taking it?"

Slowly, the reality of the situation began to hit me. "No," I answered. "What's the penalty?"

"It's a four-year suspension, Gordon."

"Four—that's—just, uh, no Olympics or World Championships, right?" I stumbled over my words, my palms sweating, my heart racing.

"It means no track and field, road racing or cross-country competition whatsoever," she answered.

My mind could barely register what Kathy was saying, that I had the right to be present when my "B" sample was tested to confirm the finding, that I had 28 days to appeal the ruling.

In Shock

I was in shock when I hung up the phone. And for days afterwards, I went around in a state of disbelief, I told only my ex-husband, Bradley, and four close friends, two of whom are doctors.

"They can't do that," said one physician friend. "You were sick and took the drug to get well." The other was shocked that Probenecid was still in my system three months after I stopped taking it.

The situation would consume me for months. I gained an education in the labyrinthine world of drug use in sports—how athletes do it, sometimes get away with it and try to conceal it. And how the wide-reaching net cast to catch and punish the guilty can ensnare the innocent.

No one ever voiced doubts about the facts of my case, which I admitted to from the start. Yes, I said over and over—to friends, acquaintances, family, coaches, sponsors, race directors, lawyers, reporters, doctors, pharmacologists, USATF officials and review panelists—I took Probenecid. I didn't know it was banned. I should have checked.

Lyme Disease

The April before that fateful New York City Marathon, Bradley and I had separated. As often happens to runners in stressful times, my sport became a refuge. I was training for the U.S. Olympic Trials 10,000 meters, to be held in June in New Orleans.

My training went well, and I qualified for the final. We had a week between the semi and the final, so I visited friends in Alabama and spent two days at an outdoor music festival. When I returned to New Orleans, I wasn't surprised to feel tired and headachy, but I was surprised when an easy 4-mile run the next day felt awful.

I slept 14 hours that night and couldn't get out of bed the next morning. I had a fever, a pounding headache, aching muscles, no appetite and a deep fatigue. The next day I went to the USOC medical center. I was examined and sent to a local hospital to be tested for dehydration and enzyme depletion. The tests showed nothing amiss. I was told I had the flu.

I spent the next three days sleeping, taking ibuprofen, drinking water and feeling sorry for myself. I figured the stress of my marital woes had caught up with me at the worst possible moment. I was a long shot to make the Olympic team, but I'd trained my butt off for the Trials. It wasn't fair.

I came home expecting to feel better soon, but weird things began to happen. I experienced severe pain in my jaw, which traveled down my neck and into my shoulders and back. The pain intensified and spread down my legs. At times my joints locked and hurt so badly I cried.

Running was out of the question; I could barely walk. Eating wasn't much of an option, either, thanks to my jaw pain. My fever shot up to 103, I got horrific headaches, and dim lamplight hurt my eyes. I lay in bed, terrified. This wasn't the flu.

I made an appointment to see an internist, Maurice Beer, recommended by a friend. He examined me and took blood and urine samples. Three days later, he called to tell me I had Lyme disease. Apparently, at some point during all the trail running I had done recently, I'd been bitten by a deer tick, the insect that transmits the disease.

"The good news is that we've caught it," he said. Tests for Lyme disease don't always pick it up, and many doctors don't think to test for it. Infected people can go around undiagnosed and untreated for months. The virus can invade the organs and cause permanent damage, and paralysis can result if the bones and joints are affected. I know of an infected woman who will probably spend the rest of her life in a wheelchair. A few cases of Lyme disease have led to death.

"So now what?" I asked. I felt inordinately happy to know what was wrong. It wasn't stress, it wasn't the flu; it was a real illness that I could now treat.

A Simple Treatment

"It's completely curable with antibiotics," said Dr. Beer. However, since my symptoms and blood test indicated that the virus had invaded the major organs, he recommended very aggressive treatment with two drugs, the antibiotic amoxycillin and Probenecid, a renal inhibitor that would keep the amoxycillin in my system by blocking its excretion from the kidneys.

I've thought back to this conversation so many times. At this point, a light bulb should have flashed in my head. I should have said, "I'm an elite runner and subject to drug testing. I can't take certain drugs. Any drug you prescribe I'll need to check with the U.S. Olympic Committee Drug Hotline."

But at the time, I was totally fixated on getting well. I was sick, alone and terrified that I would never be able to walk again, much less run. I couldn't wait to start the treatment. And the drugs must have been powerful drugs, because I started feeling better right away.

Needing to be with someone, I joined some friends for a weekend in Rockport, Massachusetts. Lyme disease isn't contagious, and I wanted to be surrounded by friends rather than be sick alone. When we arrived, late at night, I went and sat on the beach. I watched the moonlight on the gentle surf, and for the first time in months, I felt at peace.

On the Road to Recovery

In the following weeks, I made a dramatic recovery. I was able to coach at the Craftbury Running Camp in Vermont and even run the Stowe 8-Mile Road Race.

By the end of July, I felt fine. The pain, stiffness, fever and fatigue had disappeared. I had abundant energy and was back to my usual hectic schedule of training, coaching and writing.

Despite my recovery, Dr. Beer put me on another two-week drug course. "You really want to knock this virus out of your system," he said. Since the drugs didn't have any side effects, I complied. In mid-August I had another blood test. It showed that the Lyme virus had fallen to very low levels. I could stop taking the drugs.

I entered a 10-K and set a PR [personal record]. "What's going on?" I asked my coach, Benji Durden. He said I'd been in great shape, hadn't peaked because of my illness and had just gotten stronger with a month of rest. I ran a 20-K PR and was selected to run for the U.S. team at the IAAF [International Association of Athletics Federations] World Half-Marathon Championship in England on September 20. There I ran another PR, by 2 minutes.

The race confirmed my decision to run the New York City Marathon. Although Benji suggested I consider an easier course, I was set on New York. I'd done a lot of soul-searching over whether I should stay in Manhattan after ending my marriage. It's a tough place to be single, not to mention train as an elite runner. But it was home. Running the marathon would affirm my decision.

I did leave for four weeks of training in Boulder, Colorado. I wanted to spend time with Benji, who lives there, and train at altitude. My sisters, Anne and Julie, also live in Boulder, and it was wonderful to have an excuse to visit. That month I trained, slept, ate, finished an overdue book manuscript and caught up on years of conversations with Anne and Julie.

I flew home the week before the marathon, knowing I was as fit as I could be. The course and conditions were tough, and I realized early that my goal of a sub-2:30 was more than I had in me that day. I hung on for sixth place in 2:33:26, just off my PR.

Standard Procedure

"I'm with the U.S. Olympic Committee Drug Control Program," a voice behind me said, seconds after I crossed the finish line.

I went through the familiar process of producing a urine sample and pouring it into two sterile beakers marked A and B. Then I filled out the drug form. Under "List each medication used recently," I listed the iron, vitamin C and folic acid supplements I took every day. It never occurred to me to list the drugs prescribed for Lyme disease, which I'd stopped taking months earlier. And that was the last I thought about my drug test until Kathy Presnal called two weeks later.

After I absorbed the shock of the news, I reviewed my options. I could fly to Los Angeles to watch while my B sample was tested, but what was the point? The same urine was in both beakers. After reviewing USATF rules on drug-use violations, which precluded me from arguing in an appeal that the drug was prescribed by a doctor, I waived my right to appeal the finding. An athlete can appeal a positive drug test only if he or she believes the finding is incorrect. Butch Reynolds, the 400-meter world record holder who was banned by the IAAF in 1990 after testing positive for an anabolic steroid, appealed because he believed the sample tested was not his.

My final option was to apply to USATF for reinstatement. My application would be reviewed by a three-person panel selected from the National Amateur Board of Review. The panel would recommend that USATF either uphold, shorten or overturn the suspension. If they recommended the second or third option, the Executive Committee would review the case and decide. In the meantime, I had to return my prize money, I couldn't race, and I lost my USOC health insurance.

Recruiting Allies

I worked hard to put together a strong reinstatement request. I gathered as much information as I could about Lyme disease to show how ill I'd been. Dr. Beer wrote a letter supporting me, and other physicians attested to the disease's ability to impair cognitive functioning—the ability to think straight. I asked prominent people in the running community to write character references. And I asserted my adamant opposition to the use of performance-enhancing drugs. "I am committed to absolute fairness in athletics and would sooner be banned for life than ever seek any type of unfair advantage over other athletes," I wrote.

Many people helped and supported me, but others had no idea what was going on. "When's your next race, Gordon?" they'd ask. I gave vague replies.

I tried to maintain some sense of humor. I asked a friend who worked at the New York Road Runners Club for a 1996 New York City Marathon T-shirt. I flexed my skinny arms and called myself the world's weakest steroid user.

USATF publicized my suspension in a press release sent to news organizations around the country. I got 30 calls the day of the announcement and stopped answering my phone.

I wanted to be left alone. But when I was by myself, I felt panicky. I didn't want to run, but I felt lost without it. My friends would drag me out of my apartment to run and socialize.

I desperately missed being a competitive runner. I cried watching a race in Central Park. I wanted to be training for a spring marathon and thinking ahead to the 1993 World Championships.

The Hearing

My hearing was set for January 11. It was to be a telephone conference call with the three panelists, an attorney representing USATF, Dr. Beer and me. I chose not to have a lawyer represent me, feeling I'd seem less defensive representing myself.

The morning of the hearing I went for a run. No matter what happens, I thought, I still have this. I can go out on a beautiful winter morning and move my body, feel the sun on my face and the wind in my hair. I came home and put on [music by] R.E.M., sang at the top of my lungs and danced with my cat, Scout. I tried to relax enough to practice reading my statement.

When the call came, I felt focused and alert. I summarized everything that had happened to me since the Trials. I told the panel I'd never taken performance-enhancing drugs and would never dream of doing so. I said I'd suffered enough, that the prospect of a four-year suspension made my heart sink. I urged them to amend the punishment to fit the crime.

The USATF lawyer presented an open-and-shut case. Rules are rules, he said. There was no question at all that I had broken the rules and therefore should be punished accordingly.

The panelists asked lots of questions. They wanted to know why I hadn't checked with the USOC Drug Hotline. They asked Dr. Beer about alternative treatments for Lyme disease. He said they exist but are less effective when the virus has become systemic, and that they have side effects and can be very expensive.

Both the panelists and Dr. Beer wanted to know how much Probenecid was found in my urine. The USATF lawyer said that was irrelevant. A banned drug had been found; a doping violation had occurred.

Back and forth the questions fired, for almost 2 hours. When it was over, I was exhausted and drenched in sweat. I felt the conference had ended with many questions unanswered, and the questions made me see that there was more at issue here than just my honesty and intentions.

One of the panelists, a former high jumper, couldn't understand why I hadn't checked with the USOC Hotline. I felt as if she were saying: "Look, drug use is a big problem in our sport. If you don't check before taking something, you're either stupid or naive or you just don't care." I learned that some athletes take the banned-drug list with them every time they see a doctor and have the USOC Drug Hotline phone number memorized.

Tough Choices

The panelists decided we needed another hearing, which we had on January 29. It was shorter and more focused on alternative treatments for Lyme disease. Dr. Beer said the only other treatment he would have felt comfortable with was intravenous antibiotics, which would have cost $12,000 to $15,000 and required a month in the hospital.

I did a lot of thinking after that hearing. I wondered what I would have done if I had checked and found that Probenecid was banned. I decided I didn't regret anything. Taking Probenecid had helped me recover quickly and fully from a severe illness. I hadn't cheated, I hadn't hurt anyone. Once I realized these things, my life started to fall back into place. I started running more consistently, revived my social life, lined up interesting work and even interviewed for a job. I'd done all I could about my suspension—now I just had to wait.

My life turned upside down again when my mother had a heart attack on February 13. I spent most of the rest of the month with her and my dad. I hardly thought about my suspension. Then I was offered a job as health editor of *Woman's Day* magazine, which I accepted. It felt great to focus on something positive at last.

On March 1, I called Kathy Presnal to find out what was taking so long. She had just received the panel's decision: My reinstatement request had been denied.

I refused to believe it until I saw the document, which finally arrived on March 10. The decision was unanimous, based on the fact that I admitted taking Probenecid, that it was my responsibility to have called the USOC Hotline and that alternative treatments for Lyme disease exist.

That week, my mother had an angioplasty, I was preparing to start my new job, and the blizzard of '93 hit. I didn't run for nine days.

Is It Better to Admit Defeat?

Who needed running? I closed out my USATF trust account and gave away my old national team uniforms. Friends urged me to fight the decision, but I told them to leave me alone. Hadn't I had enough stress this year?

Still, the decision rankled me. I felt it was dead wrong and showed a sport that had become so paranoid about drug use that it had lost all compassion. No runner should be kicked out for four years because she made an innocent mistake.

When I read that Ben Johnson had been banned for life for his second doping offense, the injustice of my suspension hit me like the blow of a sledgehammer. Johnson had cheated; I'd made a mistake. Yet our sport had tarred us both with the same brush. I decided I didn't want to wait to right this wrong.

Fixing the System

Thanks to a provision in the USOC Constitution, I could request a hearing before the American Arbitration Association [AAA]. I hated the thought of doing this. It would be expensive, time-consuming and confrontational. Full of mixed feelings, I retained an attorney, Edward G. Williams. Ed had competed in the 1968 Olympics as a biathlete and served as the USOC's Athletes' Advisory Council chair and as chair of the USOC Legislation Committee. He'd also defended runners in the Athletes' Rights disputes in the 1970s and '80s.

He felt I had a strong case, and as we prepared for the hearing, my confidence grew, too. In fact, I became so confident that I decided to train for the Advil Mini-Marathon on June 12. I had run this women's 10-K almost every year since 1980, and I certainly didn't want to miss it this year. As I trained and coached other runners, I kept my goal a secret, in case it didn't work out.

In the end, we never had the AAA hearing. Instead, two days before the scheduled hearing, the reinstatement panel amended their decision and recommended immediate reinstatement. The Executive Committee approved the decision. Ed called with the good news on June 8. I could run in the Mini!

That my suspension was over didn't fully hit me until the morning of the race. As I walked toward the starting line, I was filled with that wonderful, intoxicating rush that comes at the start of a race. I felt the lightness of my racing flats, the heat coming off the pavement, the jumpiness in my gut, the twitchy strength in my body, the toughness in my mind. I'd missed it so much, this sense of being fully alive and in the present moment.

If anything good has come out of all of this, it's that I'll never again take competitive running for granted. I'd also like to work with the USATF to find ways to protect other athletes from an experience like mine. I'm not angry. I believe everyone did what he or she felt was best for the sport, given the current system. But clearly, it's a system that needs some work.

Let 'Em Eat Steroids

Jennifer Sey

As Jennifer Sey notes in the following essay, which was originally published during the 2008 Summer Olympics, elite athletes in sports like gymnastics and swimming often go to extreme lengths to achieve their best performance. These measures can involve using the latest high-tech equipment, going on intensive diet or exercise regimens for weight loss or gain, masking—and sometimes exacerbating—injuries by using (approved) painkillers, and sometimes by using banned performance-enhancing drugs.

Here, Sey raises legitimate questions about how and where officials, athletes, and the general public draw the line about which methods are acceptable. Sey, a former competitive gymnast, freely admits that when she was at the height of her competitive career, she would have gone to virtually any lengths if she had been assured that doing so would help improve her performance. She compares elite athletes to members of a cult, so dedicated to their cause that they are unable to make good or rational decisions.

Sey won the 1986 U.S. Gymnastics Nationals. Following a series of debilitating injuries and growing disillusionment with the sport, however, she retired soon after. She is now a vice president of global marketing for Dockers and the author of Chalked Up: Inside Elite Gymnastics' Merciless Coaching, Overzealous Parents, Eating Disorders, and Elusive Olympic Dreams.

American gymnast Shawn Johnson isn't suspected of drug use, but her super-springy floor mat artificially enhances performance.

If someone had offered me performance-enhancing drugs when I was competing as a gymnast in the 1980s, I would

Jennifer Sey, "Let 'Em Eat Steroids," *Salon*, August 10, 2008. Copyright © 2008 Salon .com. This article first appeared in Salon.com, at http://www.salon.com. An online version remains in the Salon archives. Reprinted with permission.

have taken them. If we're going to be quite literal about the phrase "performance-enhancing drugs," I did take them.

I gobbled Advil [ibuprofen] like M&Ms. True, these over-the-counter painkillers aren't on the banned-substance list. But considering that I could barely walk when entering the gym each day and I was transformed upon swallowing my first six pills, it could be argued that my performance was indeed enhanced by these capsules.

Between my left ankle, which was swollen beyond recognition and traumatized with floating bone chips, and my right leg, barely healed from a cracked femur, I had no good leg to rely on. Add to that the shin splints that attacked both legs below the knees, and I was walking wounded.

The first handful of pills usually wore off around the time I finished tumbling, at which point I had to move on to vault practice. Off to the bathroom for another four pills. This second batch never quite had the same numbing effect as the first half-dozen. But I limited myself to 10 each day, an arbitrary number that seemed somehow reasonable to me.

Going to Extremes

When the Walgreen's-variety painkillers stopped working, my doctor gave me a prescription for something stronger. A few of these choking horse pills and I was good to go. They worked so well at first, I thought I was healed and set the pills aside one hopeful day before workout. I realized no healing had occurred when I found myself limping down the vault runway, dragging each sorry leg behind the other, never picking up any decent momentum, landing in a heap with my face smashed into the ground on the other side of the horse.

Eventually the prescription meds stopped working too. On to monthly cortisone shots. These helped the fraying ankle for a time. Quelled the swelling, eased the pain. After six months of injections, they failed to extinguish the ache, reduce the grotesque distortion. I continued regardless, fearful that without them my legs might just fall off.

I also took piles of laxatives in the herculean battle to keep my weight below 100 pounds, my body fat below 3 percent.

While these surely wouldn't qualify as performance enhancers—*you* try sticking a double back when you've had four choco-flavored Ex-Lax tablets the night before—it's an indication that I would've done anything I thought might contribute to best-in-class performance. And many of the girls in my gym were doing the exact same things. We traded tips on purging like housewives trading recipes.

All That Matters Is Winning

When athletes compete at the highest levels, all that matters is winning. The environment can become cultlike, in that normal standards no longer apply. There weren't other kids in my high school who willingly shot themselves up with steroid hormones to compete in the upcoming nationals. But my coaches encouraged it, the doctor offered it, and many of my teammates lined up right behind me. It was ordinary.

I would have done anything that would have allowed me to perform better. If someone had said to me, "Bend over. Try this. It will make you stronger and faster," my leotard would have been pulled up into a wedgie to make way for the magic before Dr. Mengele [notorious Nazi physician] could have loaded up the syringe.

Michael Sokolove wrote in *Play*, the *New York Times* sports magazine, that "what's lost when drugs permeate sport is quite simple: authenticity and believability." While Shawn Johnson, America's hope for a gold in gymnastics, most certainly isn't taking steroids, she enjoys the assistance of a super-springy floor exercise mat when she performs her double twisting double back opener.

Does the helpful equipment make this feat any less believable? I don't think so. I know this enhancer seems acceptable because it doesn't put the athlete's health in danger, but by Sokolove's argument it creates a certain artificiality nonetheless.

I don't blame the athletes like Marion Jones for juicing their performance with a little extra oomph. She's caught up in her sport; she needs that little somethin' somethin' to maintain her edge. Everyone else is doing it. If you shot me up with whatever she had, I wouldn't be the fastest woman alive. It was still her out there on that track. Just as it's Shawn Johnson flipping and spinning on the floor mat.

If the athletes are willing to risk their health—which many do already without taking steroids—let them. It doesn't ruin it for me.

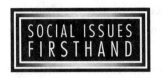

CHAPTER 3

Performance-Enhancing Drugs Outside the Arena

The Adderall Advantage

Kevin LaPorte

As teachers, students, and administrators know well, the use of performance-enhancing drugs is no longer confined to the stadium or the arena. Instead, a new generation of so-called smart drugs are becoming increasingly popular on high school and college campuses. Drugs normally prescribed for attention-deficit/ hyperactivity disorder (ADHD), such as Ritalin and Adderall, serve to boost attention spans and improve memory during cramming sessions when used by students who do not suffer from attention disorders. Drugs such as Provigil, originally meant to alleviate the sleep disorder narcolepsy, and other drugs for Alzheimer's and Parkinson's diseases are being used to improve memory and even IQ.

In the following column, originally published in the student newspaper for Loyola Marymount University in Los Angeles, the author decided to test the effects of the stimulant Adderall as he prepared to study for finals. As he reports, it was surprisingly easy to obtain Adderall, and once he started taking it, he was able to concentrate for up to eight hours of uninterrupted study. He notes, however, that there are negative side effects and worries about college students depending on it to keep up with the competition.

LaPorte is a recent graduate of Loyola Marymount University in Los Angeles, where he majored in political science.

I was somewhere around the edge of the Hannon [Library] parking lot when the drug began to take hold. I remember thinking something like "Man, I gotta get to the library . . . fast." A sudden rush of hypersensitivity and I couldn't stop staring at the individual blades of grass on Hannon field or

Kevin LaPorte, "Fearing and Loathing a Pill," *Los Angeles Loyolan*, April 23, 2007. Copyright © 2007 Los Angeles Loyolan. All rights reserved. Reproduced by permission.

counting the fronds on the palm trees along Alumni Mall. My head was buzzing and my heart was pounding out of my chest. Finals time was approaching and I knew I'd get into this rotten drug Adderall sooner or later. It was the week before finals and I had become a raving lunatic, an addict who calls in favors from friends just to get his hands on this miracle study drug.

Adderall is a prescription drug for ADHD [attention-deficit/hyperactivity disorder], something I do not have, yet nothing else mattered to me besides getting this fix. I will scratch and claw like a wild animal, I will eat my young, anything just to get the unprescribed 20 milligrams needed for an eight-hour study bender.

Not Hard to Find

Obtaining the drug was easy. A quick search through my cell phone directory for the more "jittery" of my acquaintances, a brief haggling over the $5 price and see you later! I will be a normal human being again only after I turn myself into a World Politics machine and reorganize my iTunes. There is nobody more self-serving and one-track-minded than a student in the depths of an Adderall binge. I tried to find a safe spot in the library where I hoped nobody would ruin my buzz and cause me to spiral downward into a meaningless, eight-hour study session on Facebook. I knew that possibility was very real. The slightest provocation or interruption would have been fatal to my drug-induced focus.

I found a nook on the top floor of the library with little traffic and a good view of a white wall. I cracked my books open to begin studying and ... ahh bliss! Vindication! There was nothing in the world I would rather be doing than reading about the causes of World War II. This was where I wanted to be, right there amongst my good friends Joseph Stalin and Adolf Hitler.

From outside my history bubble someone tapped my shoulder and asked, "What are you studying for?" Outrage! Blasphemy! Who would dare interrupt my concentration? I snapped around in my seat and gave my rude intruder a curt answer, then turned back to my books. But my momentum was lost. I started thinking about the moral implications of abusing this drug to get good grades. Have I really made such a beast of myself just so I can get ahead in life? I won't be sleeping or eating for the next few days—powerful side effects from the addiction.

"Every Advantage"

Our parents' generation had speed as a study drug.

Now I am taking a drug which has Amphetamines and all the same components of drug addiction. Am I really dying to use this drug? 20 children in Canada have died since 1994, causing the country to ban Adderall. The National Institute of Drug Abuse reported in 2006 that there is a 5.6 percent rate of usage amongst students on the more competitive college campuses in America. I would say that LMU [Loyola Marymount University] definitely falls under this category and I would venture to guess that our Adderall usage is much higher than 5.6 percent judging by the abundance of students with Adderall prescriptions and the ease with which I can obtain the drug.

Some would say that using Adderall is "cheating," like professional athletes who take steroids or Bob Marley smoking pot before recording a song. But nowadays you have to use every advantage you can. Adderall is the American Dream in action; anyone who is smart enough to get their hands on it will quickly rise to the top. If you don't utilize it as a scholastic weapon you'll get thrown to the wolves. Who can study straight for eight hours on their own anyways? Sooner or later, your hand will mechanically click on the scroll bar and before you know it, you will be off of ERes [electric reserves] and on to YouTube. You will have completely lost control.

I had never taken Adderall before this year. I wanted to write an article on the drug but first I needed to experience the effects before pretending to have any knowledge about Adderall. I worry about the ramifications of a college culture that uses Adderall to enhance studying methods. I hope that the next time I sit down to study I won't have some powerful Adderall craving that causes me to relapse.

Wake Up, Little Susie

David Plotz

One of the areas targeted for the application of smart drugs is Americans' chronic lack of sleep. As David Plotz points out in the following essay, millions of Americans suffer from chronic sleep deprivation. For many, caffeine is the drug of choice to help them stay awake, but its side effects include jitteriness, irregular heartbeat, and addiction. The drug modafinil (brand name Provigil) has been targeted by the U.S. military and others as a potential means to improve cognitive performance in sleep-deprived individuals without caffeine's downsides.

Plotz, the father of a young child, decides that he is a perfect candidate to try out the drug. In his experiment, he took doses of modafinil for three days and kept a diary to see how the drug affected his mood and performance. Plotz's experience certainly highlights the allure of the drug, but the author also urges caution, especially given that the drug is so relatively new and all its side effects are not yet known.

Plotz is a journalist and the editor of Slate, *an online magazine. His writings have appeared in the* The New York Times Magazine, Harper's, Reader's Digest, Rolling Stone, The New Republic, *and* GQ. *Plotz is also the author of two books, including* Good Book: The Bizarre, Hilarious, Disturbing, Marvelous, and Inspiring Things I Learned When I Read Every Single Word of the Bible.

On most days, my accumulated sleep deficit and post-lunch stupor gang up on me around 2 p.m., and I begin my slow fade. My eyes droop. Saliva dribbles onto my sweater. If I were trying to write this sentence at 2 p.m. on a normal day, it would read something like: "If I were tryyyyyyyyyyyyyyyyy . . ."

But today, I am bright-eyed and bushy-tailed, a chatty Kathy with my officemates, eager to spend all afternoon banging on the keyboard. (I normally prefer chewing my fingers off to writing.) I am not exactly wired, but I'm more alert, more focused, more Plotz-like. Today I am my own Superman, dosed on 100 milligrams of modafinil.

Every year, we need the same amount of sleep, and every year we get less. Since the invention of artificial illumination, sleep has been a bear market. There are many reasons we catch fewer Z's: Round-the-clock workplaces, longer commutes, brighter lights, 24-hour Krispy Kreme stores, the Home Shopping Network—the list goes on. According to University of Pennsylvania professor of psychology David Dinges, Americans probably sleep about six and a half to seven hours per night, compared to the more than eight hours our bodies want.

We have learned to cope with a regular sleep deficit, but we pay a price (and not just $4.05 for the venti [Starbucks' largest drink size] latte). Studies by Dinges and military scientists have proved that performance deteriorates when you sleep less than eight hours. People who rest seven or six or five hours a night may not feel tired, but their thinking and dexterity are suffering. We medicate ourselves with caffeine, a drug that raises alertness but at a cost of jitteriness, irregular heartbeat, and addiction. Folks who really need to stay awake dope themselves with amphetamines—stimulants that can ward off sleep for days but cause terrible crashes when they wear off. (And we don't know what long-term damage they cause.)

Can We Live Without Sleep?

The military is enthralled with the possibility of doing away with shut-eye. The supersecret Defense Advanced Research

Projects Agency is investigating drugs that would keep soldiers awake for a week. The Air Force prescribes "go pills"—small doses of the amphetamine Dexedrine—to pep up long-haul pilots. (But hopped-up pilots may be dangerous: The American pilots who accidentally bombed and killed Canadian soldiers [in 2002 in Afghanistan] were taking go pills.)

Avoiding sleep for a week might be necessary in an extreme situation like war, but the run-of-the-mill, office-working, wannabe Superman requires something different. We don't want a pill that will keep us Exceling and Power Pointing for three days straight. We just want something that makes us feel alert through an entire normal day—a drug that makes us feel as lively for the 18-hour-day we *have* to live as for the 16-hour-day we *ought* to live.

Hence my rendezvous with modafinil. The drug, made by Cephalon, is marketed under the creepy, pharma-Orwellian name Provigil. The FDA [Food and Drug Administration] approved it in 1998 to treat narcolepsy, but it is starting to have an underground life as a pick-me-up for the routinely sleep-deprived. The military has tested it heavily, particularly on pilots.

How Stimulants Work

The way modafinil works is not understood. It seems to slow the release of GABA, a sleep promoter in the brain. It also may act on the histamine system, which is connected to sleep regulation. What *is* clear is that modafinil differs from most other pick-me-ups, which tend to be indiscriminate in their function. Amphetamines like Dexedrine, for example, promote wakefulness by interfering with uptake of the neurotransmitter dopamine, causing dopamine to flood the brain. Dopamine, says Joyce Walsleben, director of the NYU Sleep Disorders Center, is a "broad hitter" that sets the heart racing, causes twitchiness, and makes you feel high. When the effect of such stimulants wears off, the crash is nasty. Caffeine affects a different pathway, involving adenosine, but that, too, spills over the brain's flood wall, making coffee drinkers jittery.

But modafinil tiptoes around dopamine, confining its activity to the particular neurological processes connected to wakefulness. It doesn't seem to act as a broad stimulant. (This is one reason, Walsleben says, that modafinil has not become a street drug. Unlike cocaine or amphetamines, modafinil doesn't make you feel high, and it acts very slowly, taking a couple of hours or more to kick in.) Narcoleptics seem to love modafinil. (By boosting alertness throughout the day, modafinil reduces the narcoleptic's compulsion to nod off.) Now doctors are getting barraged by requests from regular folks who want to use it to cut down on sleep.

The seduction of modafinil is that you can feel as peppy after six hours sleep as you would after nine. Doctors see modafinil as an occasional pick-me-up. They doubt you could take the drug everyday without consequences: Most sleep researchers agree that the longer sleep is necessary for hormonal regulation, among other essential bodily functions.

Tired of merely writing about enhancement (and tired, period), I decided to conduct my own unscientific trial of modafinil. As the father of a 2-year-old, I live in a constant haze of sleep deprivation. I vowed to take modafinil for a week and see what happened. Could it transform a lazy, exhausted hack into a brilliant Jeffrey Goldberg [journalist and writer]? Or recast a grouchy father into Superdad? I persuaded my doctor—and no, you can't have his number—to prescribe me a week's supply of Provigil, seven 200-milligram pills.

Here is the diary I kept.

Day 1, Monday

6:45 a.m.: Woken up by my daughter after the usual six and a half hours.

7 a.m.: I open the bottle. The pills are monstrous. I start to chicken out. I've never smoked pot, much less taken co-

caine or amphetamines. I decide to halve the dosage. When I cut the first pill with my pocketknife, half of it shoots off my bureau, slides across the floor, and disappears under a dresser, no doubt to be discovered and eaten by my daughter someday in the near future. I pop the other 100-milligram half.

10 a.m.: At the office. I've felt no rush, but alertness has snuck up on me. I am incredibly attentive, but not on edge. I really, really feel like working, a rare sensation.

12 p.m.: I reach for my usual lunchtime Coca-Cola, then think better of it. Caffeine plus this sprightliness and I will be ping-ponging off the walls.

2 p.m.: This is when I usually fold. Today I am the picture of vivacity. I am working about twice as fast as usual. I have a desperate urge to write, to make reporting calls, to finish my expense account—activities I religiously avoid. I find myself talking very loudly and quickly. A colleague says I am grinning like a "feral chipmunk."

6 p.m.: Annoyed to have to leave the office when there is all this lovely work to do.

9 p.m.: Home. After dinner, I race upstairs to start working again. This is totally out of character, especially on a *Monday Night Football* evening.

12 a.m.: I want the day to keep going but force myself to go to bed. I fall asleep easily enough, but it's a weird night. I have lots of dreams, which is unusual. All are about Getting Things Done.

Day 2, Tuesday

6:30 a.m.: I wake up feeling good, cut another pill in two, and pop a half.

9 a.m.–7 p.m.: I work like a fiend again. These have been the two most productive days I've had in years. Idea for new Provigil ad slogan: "Bosses' Little Helper."

1 a.m.: Again I'm alert through the late evening—so alert that I infuriate my wife by chattering at her long past her bedtime. This time, when I do conk out, I sleep deeply.

Day 3, Wednesday

7 a.m.: My one-man clinical trial starts to fall apart. Everyone says modafinil is not addictive, but I wake up worried about how long my supply will last. I count the pills and realize I have only five and a half left. That's just an 11-day supply. I remember that I offered a sample to a friend yesterday. I am annoyed—one day less for me. I start to cut up the remaining pills, wondering if I can divide them into thirds instead of halves.

I realize that maybe I can find a different supplier. I log onto the Internet to see if I can get modafinil on the sly. I find it cheap at the Discount Mexican Pharmacy. I feel delighted and relieved. Then I feel terrified that I am delighted and relieved. "Discount Mexican Pharmacy"?!

7:30 a.m.: I end my experiment after two days. I am acting like a lunatic. I stash the remaining pills in a distant corner of the medicine cabinet. I calm myself with the reminder that I have 11 more great days to look forward to.

So is modafinil a drug for future superpeople? Maybe. There are good reasons for doubt, though. The drug is approved only for treating narcolepsy, and doctors are not going to prescribe it like aspirin anytime soon. Though patients don't seem to get addicted to modafinil or to build a tolerance, according to Walsleben, the drug has been in use for only 10 years, and no one knows for certain that it's safe over the long term. (Cephalon and other drug companies, incidentally, are working on even more powerful wakefulness drugs, but none is on the market yet.)

I loved taking modafinil for two days. I worked supernaturally hard and well. But I'd be afraid to make it a habit. I'll use it again for a special occasion—when I am late for a deadline, perhaps. In the meantime, I'll just yawn my way through the midafternoon.

Two Days on Smart Drugs

Joanne Chen

As Joanne Chen points out in the following essay, many high-achievers like her who would never have dreamed of taking recreational drugs, drinking alcohol heavily, or even smoking cigarettes, have few, if any, qualms about using cognitive-enhancing drugs to help improve their intellectual, academic, or professional performance. Chen mentions that the drug modafinil (brand name Provigil) has, in fact, become known in academic circles as "Professor's Little Helper" because of its usefulness for clarifying thinking and improving performance during lectures. Chen wonders whether there is a double standard, as critics chastise athletes for cheating when they use steroids but look the other way when white-collar workers use prescription drugs (often obtained illegally or prescribed for off-label uses) to improve their own performance.

For her article, Chen decided to take Provigil for a limited period. She mentions that the drug not only helped her concentrate on important work but also enabled her to tackle mundane tasks. Ultimately, though, her qualms over taking drugs of any kind, and her physical reaction to this drug in particular, prompted Chen to have second thoughts about making her short-term experiment a long-term lifestyle choice.

Chen is a writer and editor living in New York City. Her work has appeared in Marie Claire, Vogue, The New York Times, *and* Life. *She is also the author of* The Taste of Sweet: Our Complicated Love Affair with Our Favorite Treats.

I would have made the perfect poster child for the "Just Say No" campaign. Black coffee—lots of it—is my only vice. I militantly oppose tobacco, sleeping pills, and excessive alcohol.

Joanne Chen, "Can A Pill Make Your Smarter?" *Marie Claire*, vol. 15, December 2008, pp. 169–71. Copyright © 2008 Hearst Communications. Reproduced by permission.

I assert a defiant No! to marijuana, cocaine, and steroids (not that anyone has ever offered me any). Somehow, I made it through prep school and college among the most prudish of friends. To me, anyone who engaged in chemical enhancements was a slacker or a cheater, and most certainly someone I didn't know.

But then I discovered Smart Drugs. Crack for nerds.

Smart Drugs, or more precisely, cognitive enhancers, include a variety of controlled substances, available—if you insist on being legal about it—only by prescription. They include stimulants such as dextroamphetamine (sold as Dexedrine and Adderall) and methylphenidate (Ritalin Concerta) for treating attention deficit hyperactivity disorder (ADHD). By mimicking the brain neurotransmitters norepinephrine and dopamine, stimulants leave you utterly consumed with the task at hand until mission accomplished. Then you're fired up to tackle something else, anything else, from organizing your sock drawer to grooming your cat.

Smart Drugs also include a class known as eugeroics, meaning "good arousal"—which for a worker bee like me, means the sort of high one gets when the mind is so crystal clear that one is able to dash off half a dozen lucid memos to the boss before 8:30 a.m. The eugeroics modafinil and armodafinil (sold as Provigil and Nuvigil) treat narcolepsy and "excessive sleepiness" (ES) due to shift work and sleep apnea. But prescribed off-label, they've also been found effective for ES due to overbearing superiors, perfectionist tendencies, and not enough hours in the day. They work by inhibiting the brain chemicals that cause fatigue, which in turn energizes the brain circuits. The outcome is alertness and, according to recent studies, focus and short-term-memory enhancement. Some say they move you from one challenge to the next with more ease than caffeine—without the jitters.

According to a reader survey conducted by the scientific journal *Nature*, one in five respondents has used prescription cognitive enhancers for nonmedical purposes—that's 50 percent more than those who reported taking these drugs for their intended use! When asked whether these practices should be allowed, 86 percent of the 1400 surveyed answered yes. Apparently, while the chattering classes tsk-tsked the doping habits of pro athletes those within their own circles—writers, designers, scientists, scholars—have been juicing up themselves, or secretly wishing they could.

In doing my own survey I was introduced to the in-house counsel of a private equity firm. He works 14- to 20-hour days and juggles 20 projects simultaneously. Tired of working late without getting the work done by quitting time, he contacted a psychopharmacologist, who prescribed the stimulant Focalin. Now, he says, "I can sit and draft an agreement for the next few hours and never look up, not even to check e-mail."

The notion was enough to make me Just Say Yes.

Trying to (Over)achieve

Drugs often fuel the spirit of an era. And if weed fired up the hippies of the '70s and cocaine invigorated the high-rolling '80s now cognitive enhancers are having their moment. Today the nerds and thinkers and overachievers have earned the spotlight—Bill Gates, Al Gore, Samantha Power, sultry multitasker Angelina Jolie. Smart Drugs offer an assist as we strive to be like them.

I decide on Provigil because, I reason, with my 12- to 16-hour days, my ES is practically the result of shift work. Plus, unlike ADHD drugs, eugeroics have thus far proved to be nonaddictive. I snag a prescription, pop a 100 mg pill, and await the emergence of my inner Brontë sister.

Within an hour, things start getting interesting. I feel not simply alert but perky and dare I say, sharp. I mail out a rebate form for my new cell phone, which normally would have been lost in the black hole of my inbox. I draw up an outline for a project due weeks later. Free from the usual late-morning restlessness, I continue down my to-do list until around 2 p.m., when I realize I should probably eat something. I don't necessarily feel smarter. But I do feel more organized and in control as I throw my efforts behind the odious tasks that I'd normally put off. And that's all I need to feel like a rock star.

My experience sounds typical, says Barbara Sahakian, Ph.D., a neuropsychologist at the University of Cambridge School of Clinical Medicine. "People are very attracted to these drugs," she says—particularly in today's distracting techno-culture, where we constantly flit from TV to text to IM to Web. "It's as if we're being trained to get bored."

Is This Cheating?

Cognitive enhancers first caught Sahakian's attention a couple of years ago, when she felt sluggish before giving a lecture and a colleague offered her Provigil. That got her wondering: Who else keeps a stash? It turns out, quite a few people. One professor told her that he swallows a pill every two weeks, on days he reserves for working on "complicated thoughts." A musician pops one before talking to the press. It was Sahakian's letter to *Nature* about her findings, titled "Professor's Little Helper," that prompted the journal to conduct its own survey.

Unless a medal or multimillion-dollar sports contract is at stake, we don't see splashy headlines about chemical enhancers. ("Brain doping snags a 10 percent raise for financial analyst!" doesn't have quite the same provocative ring as a Tour de France champion on steroids.) Still, ethicists worry: Is using these drugs a form of cheating?

When poker player Paul Phillips told the *Los Angeles Times* that Adderall and Provigil helped him win an impressive (though still modest, compared to the A-Rods of the world) $2.3 million in his tournament career, there was no public outcry. But I couldn't help but be suspicious, even though he did insist he'd been diagnosed with ADHD, fair and square.

When a student told me she earned a respectable B on a 12-page paper—after popping a pill at 11 p.m. and doing all her research and writing by 8 the next morning—I felt a bit miffed. Six cups of coffee never charged me up in the same way. Is the advantage just? And what about the kid on financial aid who would never be able to afford a pill at $10 a pop?

Nevertheless, when I myself took Provigil, it felt as legit as a double espresso.

Rewards and Risks

Provigil's effects last from six to 12 hours, and my 8 a.m. dose steamrolled right into the afternoon. I was particularly impressed when I made a phone call to cancel the services of a minister who had kindly offered to perform my wedding ceremony. I had dreaded it for days—how to say no to a servant of God?—but when I had her on the phone, it was as if the heavens opened up and instilled in me fresh logic and vocabulary.

When I discovered that Smart Drugs were being targeted by the National Institute on Drug Abuse (NIDA), an agency that concerns itself with coke addicts and glue-sniffing adolescents, I felt wrongly accused. The institute recently issued a report citing that about 7 million Americans age 12 or older have used prescription drugs for nonmedical reasons. Prescriptions for stimulants rose from 5 million in 1991 to almost 35 million in 2007. As Peter Conrad, Ph.D., author of *The Medicalization of Society* and a Brandeis University sociology professor, points out, we are no longer a country of "pharmacological Calvinism," the notion that self-improvement through hard work is more righteous than through drugs. But there are clear caveats. "Stimulants, particularly Adderall, carry a risk for addiction," says NIDA director Nora D. Volkow, Ph.D. "Modafinil is too new for us to know the long-term effects. But there's always a risk without proper surveillance." The worst side effects (though rare) for these drugs include cardiac complications, severe skin rashes, even suicidal tendencies. And while today's prescription stimulants curb the adrenaline rush caused by the amphetamines of two decades ago, all-nighter aftermaths still aren't pretty. Explains one user: "I'd be up all night and do well on my exam. But the comedown sucked. I just felt really weird, and I'd get very sweaty armpits."

A Dysfunctional Way of Living?

Volkow's warnings made sense, but just saying no is tough when, in the reality you create for yourself, too much is on the line—a deadline that could make or break your career, a deal that could mean making the next mortgage payment. But the solution may hinge on a deeper issue, says University of Pennsylvania neurologist Dr. Anjan Chatterjee. Maybe the real problem is, "Is this a dysfunctional way of living? And how do you fix that?"

In a report last May [2008], the Academy of Medical Sciences predicted that a crush of no fewer than 600 cognitive enhancers will descend on the market before the century is over. Already, pharmaceutical company Shire has created a less addictive form of Adderall for adult ADHD (wink wink). And as researchers continue to improve treatments for Alzheimer's disease, students, lawyers, bankers—or those with "memory retention disorder," jokes Conrad—will be sure to experiment with them.

Perhaps the only factor keeping overachievers from OD-ing on Smart Drugs is that the body knows it has its own right of refusal. I ended my Provigil experiment after two tries because, as much as I welcomed the rush of productivity, I didn't like the upset stomach and nausea that came with it. I renewed my relationship with coffee and allowed myself a nap once in a while—though I can't promise that, should an emergency arise in the future, I won't Just Say Maybe.

No More Butterflies

Blair Tindall

*Stage fright—and the lengths to which musicians will go to con-
trol it—just might be the dirty little secret of the classical music
world. Oboist Blair Tindall, however, is well aware of the widespread prevalence of stage fright among her musician colleagues.
She herself has experienced debilitating nervousness before audi-
tions and performances, but she manages to keep her nerves under control with the use of beta blockers. Beta blockers are typi-
cally prescribed for cardiac and hypertension patients, but have
been used by musicians, actors, and public speakers since the
1960s because of their ability to block the adrenaline that causes
those familiar nervous shakes and tremors.*

*In the following essay, Tindall describes why beta blockers
are the drug of choice for managing stage fright, given their relatively low incidence of side effects. She also questions the widely
held assumption that musicians are "more noble than other
people." The use of performance-enhancing drugs—and drugs in
general—is so widespread among the general population, why
should musicians be exempt from that?*

*Tindall is a Los Angeles–based professional oboist and jour-
nalist who writes for* The New York Times, *among other publications, and is the author of* Mozart in the Jungle: Sex, Drugs,
and Classical Music. *She has performed with world-class orchestras, including the* New York Philharmonic *and the* San Francisco Symphony, *and her work can be heard on numerous film
soundtracks.*

Professional classical musicians are a glamorous, vulnerable
and largely voiceless population. They sweep on stage in
black tie and gowns, then quietly go home; often, we know al-

most nothing about their lives outside their performance. But [now in 2008] a lesser known aspect of those seemingly decorous lives has come to light, after a horn player for Simon Rattle's Berlin Philharmonic admitted to drinking before performances to calm his nerves. "You go for tranquilisers or beer," Klaus Wallendorf told a documentary film-maker. "With me it was beer. Then you drink two beers and it goes smoothly so you think you should do it all the time." The revelation has prompted further admissions, and German tenor Roland Wagenführer expressed concerns about drug abuse in the opera world. So does classical music have a drink-and-drugs problem?

Let's start with full disclosure. I am a professional musician—an oboist—and have performed with four major orchestras in the US, including the New York Philharmonic. Like many people my age (I'm 48), I've tried marijuana and Valium in the past. Today, I drink alcohol on a social basis, as well as [use] beta blockers, which are prescribed by my doctor, and which I take for performance anxiety once or twice a year.

That's not so shocking, is it? Despite my musical accomplishments, I am a normal person who addresses various challenges like anyone else. Yet some would label me a troubled substance abuser, and say that classical musicians are trying to one-up Amy Winehouse.

What's the Attraction?

First, let's dissect the effect of various drugs, and consider why classical musicians would want to take them. Alcohol, tranquilisers, marijuana, and beta blockers have dramatically different applications and effects, many of which are undesirable for musicians. Musicians are not exempt from alcoholism, and it affects performance in a negative way. Classical musicians rely on minute technique and quick response time; alcohol only dampens these skills, and although initially it might ameliorate stage fright, once on stage, drunkenness only amplifies terror. The violinist Nigel Kennedy may have a reputation as a hellraiser, but even he says he would only smoke or drink after a concert—never before. "Performing under the influence of alcohol or dope would be cheating the audience," he told *Focus* magazine in Germany. I have seen, on rare occasions, musicians drinking pre-concert, and it never works out well.

Cocaine is a drug only the most successful musicians use—because it's expensive. (Newsflash: working-class musicians don't earn big.) In small amounts, cocaine does seem to enhance confidence, which, depending on how much preparation you've put in, could be a good thing—or highly embarrassing when it comes to reading the reviews the next morning. I do know musicians who use it while performing, but they are a tiny minority.

Tranquilisers like Valium have similar consequences to alcohol: they compromise technique and response time. Still, some people are prescribed these drugs for medical reasons, so it's difficult to separate the "abusers" from the legitimate patients.

Few people use marijuana these days. In general, musicians want and need to be mentally acute. Pot doesn't fit the bill. Furthermore, one of the drug's main symptoms is paranoia, which doesn't go well with stage fright.

Beta Blockers: The Right Choice?

Finally we come to beta blockers, a class of heart medications that treat blood pressure, angina and migraines. Since a 1965 *Lancet* article explored their use for stage fright, they've also been widely prescribed for musicians, public speakers, and even surgeons who must steady their hands.

Beta blockers are not recreational drugs. They do not affect cognitive abilities, but instead block adrenaline-like chemicals in the human system. For a violinist, this means performance can feel like practice, with no bouncing bow or slippery fingers.

An article in the *Times* [of London] yesterday [June 4, 2008,] reported that there is a "black market" for beta blockers among classical musicians. But these are legal drugs—taken for medical reasons by as many as 10% of the world's (and therefore any orchestra's) population; they are routinely prescribed for stage fright.

A Miracle Cure for Stage Fright

As a teenager, I suffered debilitating stage fright. When I went to college, I asked the conducting staff to assign me to pit orchestras, instead of onstage groups. And so I asked my doctor for a prescription for beta blockers.

On the subway in New York in 1986, I took my first dose of Inderal, a beta blocker, some 45 minutes before an audition. It seemed miraculous. Although I still felt nervous, my hands didn't shake as usual, I wasn't gasping for air and my mind remained clear. I played exactly as I had meticulously prepared to do. I won the job, and went on to play a Carnegie Hall debut recital, record a Grammy-nominated CD, and hold a solo position with four major Broadway productions.

Beta blockers are not a class of drug that's subject to abuse. No one would want to overdose: I once took too much (which I later learned was only a quarter of my elderly mother's daily prescription) and the boring performance that ensued made me commit to smaller doses from then on.

Musicians Are Human, Too

It always seems surprising to audiences that classical musicians are like any other cross section of society—subject to the same joys, sorrows, and misbehaviour. Yes, some musicians are alcoholics. Some are stoners, who stumble through life on pot, middling about on the worst possible gigs, ones that barely support them. Some lose everything in the wake of cocaine and crack abuse.

I knew a beautiful blonde cellist in New York in the 1980s, who was married, owned a gorgeous apartment overlooking Central Park, and landed a chair in Phantom of the Opera, which is [still] playing two decades later. Yet she surrendered to cocaine, and then crack. She died three years ago after battling AIDS for a decade, leaving behind a young son. She was a stellar musician, but also an ordinary human being with demons like anyone else.

Three years ago, I published a book about drugs and classical music, *Mozart in the Jungle.* On my book tour, a journalist asked me to clarify why "musicians are more noble than other people". Where did he get such an idea? Although most of us don't end up in dire circumstances, we, like anyone else, are just people. We're tempted. We say yes or no to drugs. But, because of our discipline, we most often say no: drugs and impairment are not worth risking a lifetime of practice.

Organizations to Contact

The editors have compiled the following list of organizations concerned with the issues debated in this book. The descriptions are derived from materials provided by the organizations. All have publications or information available for interested readers. The list was compiled on the date of publication of the present volume; the information provided here may change. Be aware that many organizations take several weeks or longer to respond to inquiries, so allow as much time as possible.

Association Against Steroid Abuse
521 N. Sam Houston Pkwy. East, Ste. 635, Houston, TX   77060
Web site: www.steroidabuse.org

The Association Against Steroid Abuse is dedicated to providing current information about steroids to potential abusers as well as parents, teachers, and coaches. The association's Web site includes several true stories from steroid users, as well as statistics and warning signs for steroid abuse. The Web site also offers detailed information about specific steroid drugs and offers an "ask the doctor" feature and a link to informational online videos.

ATHENA & ATLAS
3181 SW Sam Jackson Park Rd., Portland, OR   97239-3098
(503) 418-4166 • fax: (503) 494-1310
e-mail: chpr@ohsu.edu
Web site: www.ohsu.edu/ohsuedu/academic/som/medicine/hpsm/center.cfm

ATHENA (Athletes Targeting Healthy Exercise & Nutrition Alternatives) and ATLAS (Athletes Training & Learning to Avoid Steroids) are programs sponsored by the Center for Health Promotion Research at Oregon Health & Science University. ATHENA (for female athletes) examines the connections among young women in sports, disordered body image, and body-shaping drug use. ATLAS (for male athletes) focuses on healthy nutrition and strength training as alternatives to steroid use. Both programs consist of multiple small-group sessions led by coaches and student team leaders. Sample program materials are available for download at the Web site.

Athletes Against Steroids

731 Kirkman Rd., Orlando, FL   32811

(877) 914-9910

e-mail: tomc@athletesagainststeroids.org

Web site: www.athletesagainststeroids.org

Athletes Against Steroids is devoted to educating amateur and professional athletes about the dangers of steroids. The organization's Web site serves as a clearinghouse of information about steroids designed to discourage use, with a list of steroid side effects, true stories written by former steroid users, links to relevant news articles and opinion pieces, and a list of athletes who have died while using the drugs. The organization publishes a free weekly e-newsletter; subscription sign-up is available on the Web site.

Bike Pure

Bavan, O'Meath, Co. Louth
  Ireland

+44 (0)7825 339011

e-mail: info@bikepure.org

Web site: www.bikepure.org

Bike Pure aims to protect the integrity of cycling and promote clean cyclesport. The organization lobbies for stiffer penalties for cyclists who violate antidoping policies and endorses cycling athletes who sign the organization's Honor Code. Bike Pure's Web site lists the teams and individual riders who have signed the Honor Code. To promote awareness, Bike Pure sells cycling jerseys and armbands and offers screen savers and mobile wallpapers for free download on its Web site.

Coalition for Anabolic Steroid Precursor and Ephedra Regulation (CASPER)

2099 Pennsylvania Ave. NW, Ste. 850, Washington, DC 20006
(202) 419-2521 • fax: (202) 419-2510
e-mail: feedback@casper207.org
Web site: www.casper207.org

The mission of Coalition for Anabolic Steroid Precursor and Ephedra Regulation (CASPER) is to influence health-care decisions by promoting healthy, healing, humane and ethical environments to positively impact the health of the public and the advancement of quality critical care. Made up of organizations in medicine, public health, and sports, CASPER lobbies for regulations on dietary supplements that contain steroid precursors and the herbal substance ephedra. The coalition's Web site offers fact sheets and sample letters that supporters can forward to their congressional representatives.

J. Kyle Braid Leadership Foundation

53634 Road NN 56, PO Box 166, Villa Grove, CO 81155
(719) 655-2270 • fax: (719) 655-2290
Web site: www.jkbranch.org

Established in memory of J. Kyle Braid, a high school athlete who took his own life while on steroids, the J. Kyle Braid Leadership Foundation educates potential peer leaders to help other students resist negative peer pressure and destructive behaviors. High school sophomores participate in the program by attending a summer workshop at a Colorado ranch. They then bring the skills they learn back to their own communities and schools. In addition to empowering teen leaders, the foundation also educates coaches on how to be positive influences in kids' lives.

The National Center for Drug Free Sport

2537 Madison Ave., Kansas City, MO 64108
(816) 474-8655 • fax: (816) 502-9287
e-mail: info@drugfreesport.com
Web site: www.drugfreesport.com

The National Center for Drug Free Sport was founded in 1999 to provide drug-testing services to sports programs nationwide. Since then, the center has expanded to provide resources and education for sports programs at all levels, from amateur to collegiate to professional. Speakers from the organization's roster present antidoping talks at colleges and universities across the country. The center's Web site offers a subscription-based resource exchange center, which provides up-to-date information about dietary supplements and dangerous and banned substances. The center's quarterly newsletter, *Insight*, is available free online.

The National Coalition for the Advancement of Drug-Free Athletics

PO Box 206, New Milford, NJ   07646
(201) 265-8688
Web site: www.ncadfa.org

The mission of the National Coalition for the Advancement of Drug-Free Athletics is to support the advancement of drug-free athletes at the national level through the continued development of educational community outreach, leadership, and drug awareness programs. The organization's motto is "True champions choose not to use." Founded in 2004, the coalition is composed of addiction specialists, sports psychologists, and other health and fitness professionals focused on educating athletes and coaches about the dangers of performance-enhancing drugs and on advocating healthier strategies for optimizing athletic performance. These experts present educational seminars for teams and schools across the country.

755 HITS

e-mail: TeamMembers@755hits.org
Web site: www.755hits.org

755 HITS is a nonprofit organization promoting the idea that any athlete who breaks a sports record by cheating (including using performance-enhancing drugs) should have his or her record invalidated. Inspired by baseball player Henry "Hank"

Aaron's lifetime home run number, the "HITS" in the organization's name also refer to "honesty, integrity, and truth in sports." The organization contributes money raised through donations to its Web site to education and awareness campaigns, especially to nonprofessional and youth sports programs that encourage fair play.

Taylor Hooton Foundation
PO Box 2104, Frisco, TX   75034-9998
(972) 403-7300
Web site: www.taylorhooton.org

The Taylor Hooton Foundation was established in honor of high school athlete Taylor Hooton, who committed suicide after developing severe depression while using anabolic steroids. Speakers from the foundation give talks about the dangers of steroids to high school assemblies and other organizations. The foundation's Web site offers several true stories of steroid abuse and recovery, as well as facts about performance-enhancing drugs and a glossary of terms. The Web site also includes a blog covering related topics in the news.

United States Anti-Doping Agency (USADA)
1330 Quail Lake Loop, Ste. 260
Colorado Springs, CO   80906-4651
(719) 785-2000 • fax: (719) 785-2001
Web site: www.usantidoping.org

The U.S. Congress recognizes the United States Anti-Doping Agency (USADA) as "the official anti-doping agency for Olympic, Pan American and Paralympic sport in the United States." Founded in 2000, this nongovernmental agency provides education and resources about doping, works to ensure that only athletes who are guilty of a doping violation are sanctioned, strives to systematically identify and sanction those individuals who are engaged in doping, and funds research to advance detection. Its Web site offers athletes, coaches, and trainers a comprehensive database of prohibited substances and information and a list of answers to frequently asked questions, as well as numerous publications about antidoping control and testing. The USADA's quarterly newsletter, *The Spirit of Sport,* is available free online.

World Anti-Doping Agency (WADA)
Stock Exchange Tower, 800 Place Victoria, Ste. 1700
PO Box 120, Montreal, Quebec   H4Z 1B7
   Canada
(514) 904-9232 • fax: (514) 904-8650
Web site: www.wada-ama.org

The World Anti-Doping Agency (WADA) was established in 1999 as a cooperative project funded by national governments and sports-governing bodies. Its key activities include scientific research, education, development of antidoping capacities, and monitoring of the World Anti-Doping Code. The code can be downloaded from WADA's Web site, as can a number of Tool Kits that enable coaches, teachers, and athletes to equip themselves with antidoping information and strategy. WADA's Web site also offers an antidoping glossary and an interactive antidoping quiz where users can test their knowledge of doping policies. WADA's official publication, *Play True,* is available for free online.

For Further Research

Books

Shaun Assael, *Steroid Nation: Juiced Home Runs Totals, Anti-aging Miracles, and a Hercules in Every High School: The Secret History of America's True Drug Addiction.* New York: ESPN, 2007.

Howard Bryant, *Juicing the Game: Drugs, Power, and the Fight for the Soul of Major League Baseball.* New York: Plume, 2006.

Jose Canseco, *Vindicated: Big Names, Big Liars, and the Battle to Save Baseball.* New York: Simon Spotlight, 2008.

Paul Dimeo, *A History of Drug Use in Sport: 1876–1976.* New York: Routledge, 2007.

Mark Fainaru-Wada, *Game of Shadows: Barry Bonds, BALCO, and the Steroids Scandal That Rocked Professional Sports.* New York: Gotham, 2006.

Caroline Hatton, *The Night Olympic Team: Fighting to Keep Drugs Out of the Games.* Honesdale, PA: Boyds Mills, 2008.

Cynthia Kuhn, Scott Swartzwelder, and Wilkie Wilson, *Pumped: Straight Facts for Athletes About Drugs, Supplements, and Training.* New York: Dover, 2000.

Nathan Jendrick, *Dunks, Doubles, Doping: How Steroids Are Killing American Athletics.* Guilford, CT: Lyons, 2006.

Anthony Roberts, *Generation S: Tales for a Steroid Culture.* Toronto: ECW Press, 2010.

Daniel M. Rosen, *Dope: A History of Performance Enhancement in Sports from the Nineteenth Century to Today.* Westport, CT: Praeger, 2008.

Michael J. Sandel, *The Case Against Perfection*. Cambridge, MA: Harvard University Press, Belknap Press, 2007.

Stanley H. Teitelbaum, *Athletes Who Indulge Their Dark Side: Sex, Drugs, and Cover-Ups*. Westport, CT: Praeger, 2009.

Ida Walker, *Recreational Ritalin: The Not-So-Smart Drug*. Philadelphia: Mason Crest, 2008.

Warren Willey, *Better than Steroids*. Bloomington, IN: Trafford, 2007.

Periodicals

V. Cakic, "Smart Drugs for Cognitive Enhancement: Ethical and Pragmatic Considerations in the Era of Cosmetic Neurology," *Journal of Medical Ethics*, October 2009.

John A. Caldwell, "Go Pills in Combat: Prejudice, Propriety, and Practicality," *Air & Space Power Journal*, Fall 2008.

Economist, "For the Joy of It," August 2, 2008.

Marifel Mitzi F. Fernandez and Robert G. Hosey, "Performance-Enhancing Drugs Snare Nonathletes, Too," *Journal of Family Practice*, January 2009.

Jason Kirby, "Going to Work on Smart Drugs," *Maclean's*, October 13, 2008.

John Leland, "For Elderly Athletes, Drug Use Is a Given, but So Are the Whispers," *New York Times*, August 19, 2009.

G. Lippi, M. Franchini, and G. Cesare Guidi, "Switch Off the Light on Cycling, Switch Off the Light on Doping," *British Journal of Sports Medicine*, March 2008.

Jack McCallum, "The Real Dope: It's Not Just Sports," *Sports Illustrated*, March 17, 2008.

Andy Miah, "Rethinking Enhancement in Sport," *Annals of the New York Academy of Science*, 2006.

James Poniewozik, "This Is Your Nation on Steroids," *Time*, December 20, 2004.

Geoffrey Rap, "Blue Sky Steroids," *Journal of Criminal Law & Criminology*, Summer 2009.

Barbara Sahakian and Sharon Morein-Zamir, "Professor's Little Helper," *Nature*, December 14, 2007.

M. Schermer, "On the Argument That Enhancement Is 'Cheating,'" *Journal of Medical Ethics*, February 2008.

Brian Schmotzer, Patrick D. Kilgo, and Jeff Switchenko, "'The Natural'? The Effect of Steroids on Offensive Performance in Baseball," *Chance*, Spring 2009.

Angela J. Schneider and Jim L. Rupert, "Constructing Winners: The Science and Ethics of Genetically Manipulating Athletes," *Journal of the Philosophy of Sport*, vol. 36, no. 2, 2009.

Joel Stein, "Cheating Rocks!" *Time*, August 17, 2009.

L. Jon Wertheim and David Epstein, "The Godfather," *Sports Illustrated*, March 17, 2008.

Alexander Wolff, "Continental Divide," *Sports Illustrated*, July 13, 2009.

Index